2295

MW01602972

THE PHYSICAL CAPACITIES EVALUATION:

ITS USE IN FOUR MODELS OF CLINICAL PRACTICE

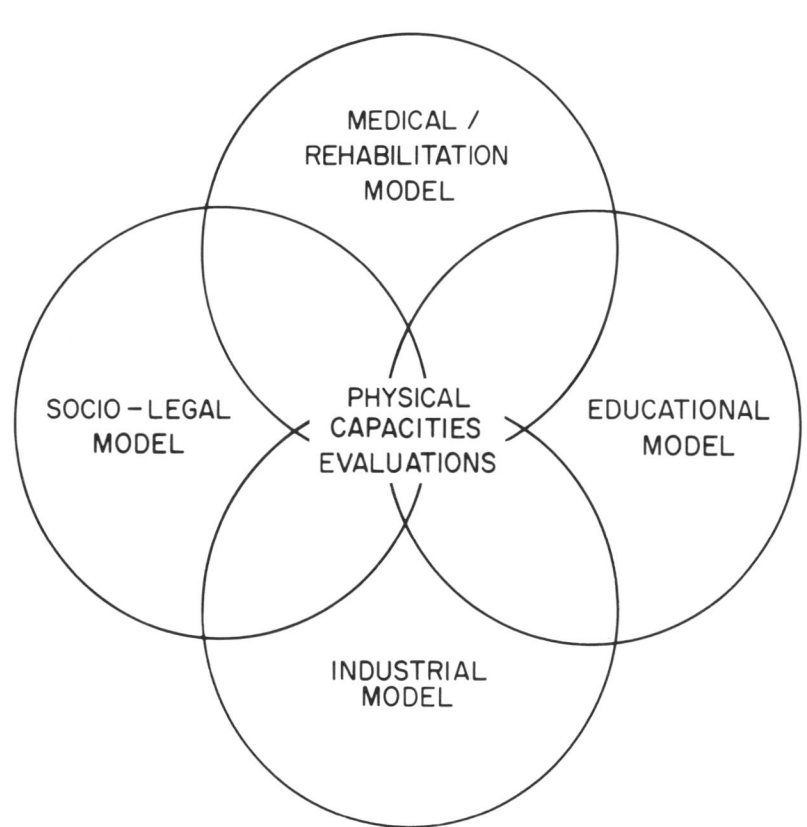

SUSAN L. SMITH, MA, OTR/L

PATRICIA BAXTER-PETRALIA, MS, OTR/L

ISBN 0-935273-02-6

Published by CHESS Publications, Inc. Business Office: 232 East University Parkway, Baltimore, MD 21218-2830

Printed in the United States of America

ACKNOWLEDGMENTS

THE AUTHORS EXTEND THEIR SINCERE APPRECIATION to those who have helped and supported their efforts to make this book a reality. Among these friends, special thanks goes to the staff at the Hand Rehabilitation Center of Philadelphia, PA, and the Professional Occupational Therapy Services, Metairie, LA, for their ongoing encouragement: Laura Bruening, Marianne Koehler, Debbie Beaulieu, Sue Blackmore for their contribution in the development of the work therapy services at the Hand Center; Teri Stahller, Marge Lloyd, Joann DiMattia, Claire McBride, Tim Powers, Kim Hunter, and Ellen McCann; Peter Fayard, Heather Meyer, Allen Dufour, Rhonda Crews, and Carla Sansone for their technical assistance; Madelyn Anderson, Anne Callahan, Florence Cromwell and Karen Stewart for their critical review and comments of the final manuscript; and to family, especially Sabastian Petralia for his cheerful and positive support throughout the writing of the book.

DEDICATION

THIS BOOK IS DEDICATED TO THE MANY occupational therapists throughout the evolution of the profession, who in the past, present, and future, will be involved with providing work-related services for their clients and patients.

PREFACE

THE UPHEAVAL CAUSED BY CHANGING NEEDS and markets in the health care industry has led to a blurring of disciplines, the emergence of new areas of specialization, and a revamping of some ideas that had become outdated. The changes wrought affect the services traditionally offered by health-related and rehabilitation disciplines. The reemergence of work-related services mandated by the consumer is central to the services of occupational therapists.

Wellness, fitness, and readiness for work are among the consumer needs now addressed by a multitude of disciplines. But these new concerns have led to a confusion regarding the roles played by disciplines with overlapping areas of expertise. Without a clear understanding on the part of the professional of the role of a discipline, the team approach has decreased value, and the consumer does not gain the optimal benefit of services. In view of this situation, the occupational therapist is finding the need to acquire new skills and to refresh skills and knowledge of work-related services.

Although known for their adaptability and creativity, occupational therapists often do not have the budget for expensive work tolerance equipment, and at times purchase equipment that is later found not as useful in treatment as anticipated. To address this problem, this book is intended to serve as a ready reference for therapists who are initiating or offering work-related services. The authors encourage the therapist to be creative and to use the physical capacities evaluation as a basis for offering and assessing work-related services. High-quality programs are possible with a low as well as a high budget. It is not necessary to have costly equipment in order to have quality. Rather, the services offered should be maximized by the use of a variety of equipment and media that will specifically meet the need of each individual who is being readied for reentry or even initial entry into the job market.

CONTENTS

CHAPTER ONE

THE THERAPIST'S ROLE AS A TEAM MEMBER

ALTHOUGH THE REHABILITATION TEAM MAY INclude individuals from numerous specialty disciplines, this book focuses on the role of the occupational therapist working on a team that includes the physician, physical therapist, and vocational evaluator. The book delineates the specialized role of the occupational therapist in this context.

Occupational therapy services are based primarily upon two frames of reference: Kielhofner and Burke's (1983) "Model of Human Occupation" and Reed and Sanderson's (1980) "Theory of Competence and Adaption of Occupational Behavior." Both models give a sound basis from which to plan treatment. For the medically impaired person, therapists intervene according to a variety of approaches to restore function and to expand capacity. By identifying a frame of reference, one can provide a more comprehensive approach to treatment.

OCCUPATIONAL THERAPY'S FRAMES OF REFERENCE VERSUS THE MEDICAL MODEL

Kielhofner and Burke's "Model of Human Occupation" provides a means of identifying and describing a patient's unique reaction to the onset of physical disability as well as the patient's needs that influence treatment planning (Kielhofner 1985). Reed and Sanderson's (1980) "Theory of Competence and Adaptation of Occupational Behavior" suggests that occupational therapists should promote maximum occupational performance through skill development that is consistent with each individual's needs. Therapists using either of these frames of reference examine in detail the components of each patient's daily requirements, including those of work and play. They also assess the actual changes in the patient's abilities, habits, roles, and environment caused by a medical impairment.

Both of these models are more comprehensive than the widely used medical model (Reed and Sanderson 1980), where the focus is on illness rather than on the needs of the individuals and their capabilities of achieving their rehabilitation potentials (Kielhofner 1985). As such, persons are evaluated on their undesirable bodily states, rather than their bodily assets.

MODEL OF HUMAN OCCUPATION

Kielhofner and Burke suggest that occupational therapists can tap the deepest and most powerful adaptive response in individuals by providing the therapeutic evaluation and intervention to facilitate those individuals' search for challenge and meaning in occupation (Kielhofner 1983). They state that occupation is not a compendium of work, rest, and play, but a necessary, dynamic, and delicate balance of daily human activities. Accordingly, individuals should be viewed as complex, open systems that interact with the environment and that maintain and change themselves through their output and performance. With a medical impairment, the physical capacities of these systems may be diminished. In order to plan effective therapeutic measures, the therapist should become aware of the extent of the disturbances in the individual that interfere with functioning in regard to roles, habits, choices, values, and interests.

Individuals who experience traumatic and permanent change in their physical situation must adjust to changes that have to be made in their everyday life. In addition to the frustrations encountered due to the loss of physical abilities, loss of roles, changes in habits and interests, and loss of control of one's schedule and choices of activities, a disabled person is also faced with changes in attitude of social groups and cultural prejudices. Family relationships may deteriorate because of the changes in roles and stress produced by the necessity to modify one's occupational behavior. People may focus on the person's limitations rather than abilities. The effect of the many changes that occur is often internalization of a negative self-esteem and an apparent lack of motivation of the medically impaired person.

THEORY OF COMPETENCE AND ADAPTATION OF OCCUPATIONAL BEHAVIOR

Reed and Sanderson state that, "The value of occupational therapy is principally in the skill of occupational therapists to examine the total performance output on an individual in terms of identifiable problems of performance" (1980, p.17). The occupational therapist evaluates an individual's competencies in three areas of occupational activity: self-maintenance, work, and play. Individuals need all three competencies in order to function at their fullest. Each individual interacts with the environment and achieves a sense of well-being by balancing the time and effort spent in each occupational activity in accordance with his or her level of competence. Competence, in turn, is achieved by balancing the time and effort spent to bring each of the skills up to a level of efficiency that is indicative of physical, psychological, and social health.

According to Reed and Sanderson, five skills are required in work, play, or self-maintenance occupational activities: motor, sensory, cognitive, intrapersonal, and interpersonal. The individual uses these skills together to produce an integrated performance.

An individual's skills can be affected by the level of educational development, by how often the skills are performed, and by the occurrence of disease, accident, or trauma. The individual's adaptive potential may be affected by intervention to reduce deficits and establish competencies in occupational performance, as well as to promote the development of skills that permit the individual to change and adapt to the changes in the environment.

The therapist can assist an individual toward change by promoting an environment that permits the development and practice of skills and by suggesting alternative skills or adaptive environments.

An individual's adaptive potential may be assessed in part by determining the degree to which the environment can be adjusted.

THE PHYSICAL CAPACITIES EVALUATION AS A RECORD OF PHYSICAL STATUS

The Physical Capacities Evaluation can be used to record each person's performance and to determine the extent to which the diminished performance has influenced roles, habits, interests, values, and self-control. Therapy should be designed to capture the individual's attention and to promote a positive morale. The environment should increase function in mental, physical, and social domains. All efforts should be focused on organized wholeness, not partial functioning or modification of pathology. The ultimate goal is to return the individual to a satisfying and useful occupational life.

IMPAIRMENT VERSUS DISABILITY

The American Medical Association (AMA) provides guides to assist physicians in rating impairments to the bodily system and in delineating their role in the work-related rehabilitation and habilitation process. AMA's *Guide to the Evaluation of Permanent Impairment* (1988) clearly differentiates medical impairment from disability. It also describes the scope of the physician's expertise and responsibilities in both of these matters. The guide provides an authoritative means for the physician to provide a clinically sound and reproducible rating of permanent impairment based upon the most advanced and comprehensive application of current medical knowledge. It distinguishes impairment ratings and degrees of disability: The impairment rating is a determination of a person's "alteration of health status assessed by physical means" whereas a disability is "that which is an alteration of the patient's capacity to meet personal, social, or occupational demands, or to meet statutory or regulatory requirements, which is assessed by non-medical means" (American Medical Association, 1988, pp. 1-2).

No assumption can automatically be made that any given disability is equivalent to any given medical impairment. The disability may be of an equal, greater, or lesser extent than the impairment. The extent of the disability must be evaluated not only medically, but also non-medically by rehabilitation professionals other than the physician.

ROLES OF HEALTH PROFESSIONALS

The physician has responsibility for the overall management of the care plan, including determining the medical impairment, if any, and outlining any medical contraindications relating to the emotional, psychological, and physical well-being of the patient.

The physical therapist focuses on restoring and maintaining muscle strength and the mobility of joints, preventing and correcting deformities, and increasing overall mobility for walking and transfer activities (Louisiana Revised Statute 37:2401 1983). The physical therapist evaluates and remediates anthropomorphic characteristics, including posture, muscle tone, strength, and joint mobility. The physical therapist also evaluates and remediates mobility status, including gait and transfer capacity.

The occupational therapist assesses physical as well as psychological needs and remediates human functioning by minimizing handicaps and maximiz-

ing functional capacities. The occupational therapist carries out these tasks with the aim of increasing the individual's functionality in both work activities and the activities of daily living.

Historically, vocational evaluators and vocational adjustment specialists have focused on evaluation of a person's psychological, intellectual, and specific aptitude skills related to the performance of work activities. These specialists contribute as a team member to the return or entry of the medically impaired person into the labor force by evaluating the person's actual and potential skills and knowledge in relation to work, and by evaluating and promoting in the individual those behavior characteristics that are necessary for success in the workplace.

In order to be cost effective and most beneficial to the patient, all of the preceding specialists should work as a comprehensive team, each providing his or her special contributions. (Figures 1, 2) In this way, the medically impaired person will have the best chance of returning or entering the labor force.

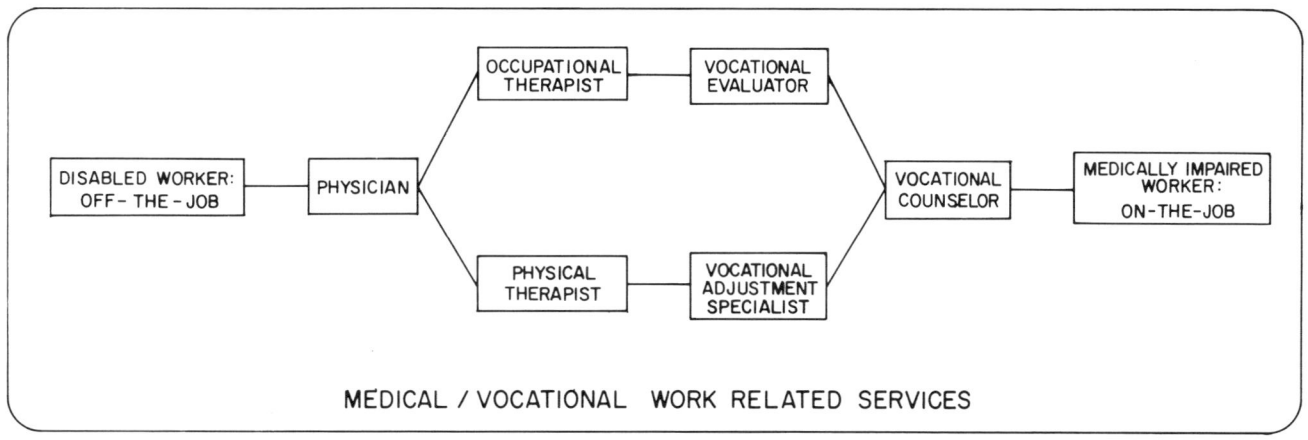

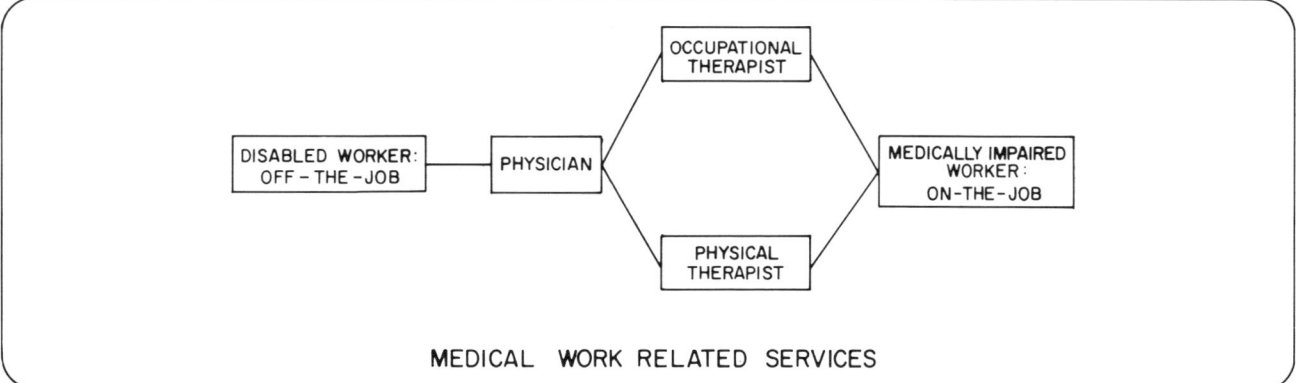

Figure 1

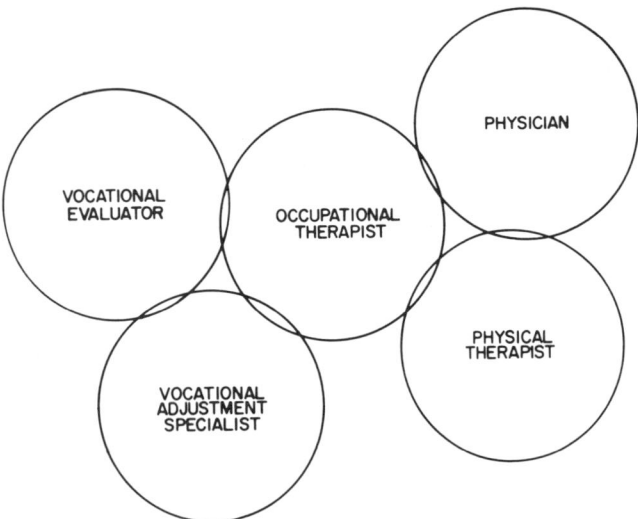

Figure 2 Overlapping roles of disciplines concerned with readying an individual for the work force.

Among the intervention models in which an occupational therapist is a team member are the rehabilitation-medical model, industrial model, educational model and legal model. (Figure 3)

Rehabilitation-Medical Model

Reduction of pathology is the short-term goal in the rehabilitation-medical model of intervention. The

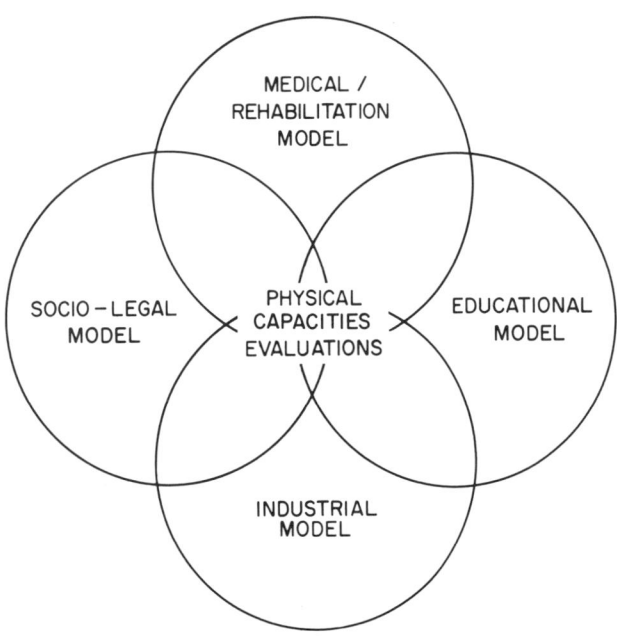

Figure 3 Four overlapping models of occupational therapy practice in which the physical capacities evaluation is used.

long-range goal is to teach the patient to adapt to his or her alternate life style which has come about because of certain residual impairments. According to this model, the therapist provides rehabilitation services in several types of facilities, including acute-care and rehabilitative centers and hospitals, specialty and general outpatient rehabilitation centers, private practices, and research centers.

Industrial Model

Occupational therapists working in industry focus on keeping workers on the job by minimizing work stresses. Their services may include consultation with employers to identify workers' physical capacities and limitations, recommendations for changes in work sites to eliminate unnecessary physical strains on workers, and the provision of management and employee education seminars. Industrial locations include outpatient facilities, industrial plants, industrial medicine clinics, and other work sites.

Educational Model

Occupational therapists became adjunct service providers for children with the 1978 Education for All Children Act (Gilfoyle, 1984, p.579). The major focus for the occupational therapist in this regard is to address students' functional deficits in order to improve their academic abilities. At junior high and high school levels, pre-work and career skills become a part of the curriculum. Services are provided in public school systems, as well as activity work centers, sheltered workshops, and group homes.

Socio-Legal Model

Medical technological advances have given longer life expectancies to the ill and disabled. Many people are injured on the job by defective products, or in accidents caused by the negligence or error of another person or a manufacturer. As the public has become increasingly aware of its legal rights, the demand for legal assistance has increased. As an expert in physical and functional evaluation, the occupational therapist can provide testimony in personal injury litigation and administrative hearings (Smith 1984). The therapist may thus serve as an expert witness in state or federal courts, or in official hearing rooms for workers' compensation or social security disability claims and other related socio-legal matters.

REFERENCES

American Medical Association. *Guides to the Evaluation of Permanent Impairment*, 3rd Ed., Chicago, 1988.

Gilfoyle, E.M. "The Eleanor Clarke Slagle Lecture, 1984: Transformation of a Profession." *American Journal of Occupational Therapy*, 38, (1985): pp. 574-84.

Kielhofner, G. and Burke, J.P. "The Evolution of Knowledge and Practice in Occupational Therapy: Past, Present, and Future." In *Health through Occupation: Theory and Practice in Occupational Therapy* (Ed. Kielhofner, G.). Philadelphia: F.S. Davis, 1983.

Louisiana Revised Statute 37:2401 (Physical Therapy Practice Act), (Sept. 1984).

Reed, K.L. and Sanderson, S.R. *Concepts of Occupational Therapy*. Baltimore: Williams and Wilkins, 1980.

Smith, S.L. "The Forensic Model of Occupational Therapy," *Occupational Therapy in Health Care*, 1 (1984): pp. 17-22

CHAPTER TWO

THE SMITH PHYSICAL CAPACITIES EVALUATION: THE PERFORMANCE COMPONENT

THE SMITH PHYSICAL CAPACITIES EVALUATION (SPCE) is designed as an objective evaluation of the way a person uses his or her body to meet the physical demands of activity. The evaluation is based on the 20 physical demands the U.S. Department of Labor (1991) specifies as possible physical demands of jobs. These demands include gross motor skills such as stooping, walking, lifting, carrying, pushing, and pulling. The evaluation may be used for analyzing a person's functional capacity for the performance of job-related, avocational, and self-maintenance activities. The results may be used for treatment planning, legal testimony, or vocational planning.

The evaluation is cost effective in its use of space and equipment and in the time required for administration, interpretation, and reporting. Other work capacities or physical capacities evaluations are frequently made over a two- to four-week period; the SPCE can be administered in one to two-and-a-half hours. Interpretation and dictation take another one to two hours. The time involved will depend in part upon the complexity of the problems presented and the skill level of the therapist. Average administration time is one to one-and-a-half hours, increasing to two-and-a-half to three hours when a functional evaluation is also administered.

TEST DESIGN

The SPCE incorporates at least one subtest for each of the 20 physical demands. Multiple subtests are used when the particular physical demand may have common variations. For example, climbing includes subtests for climbing a ramp, stair, curb, straight ladder and step-ladder (Figure 1). By contrast, crouching includes only one subtest (Figure 2).

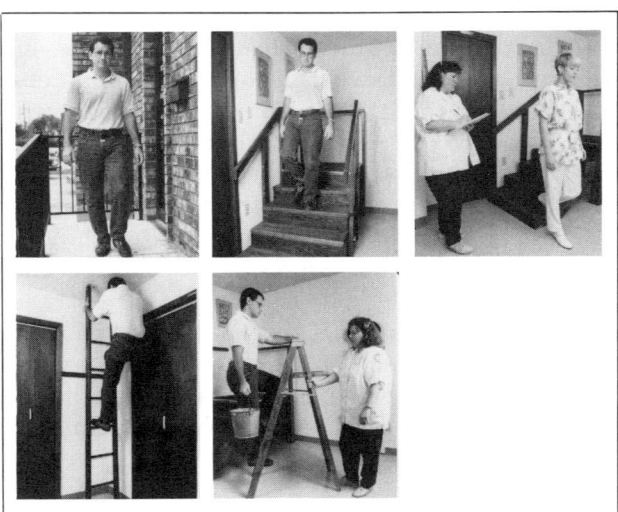

Figure 1

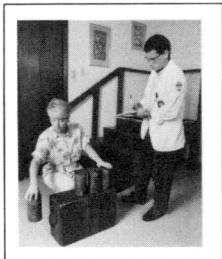

Figure 2

The subtest for walking, sitting, and standing includes a section for the patient to estimate endurance. This is particularly important when one's endurance is greater than that seen during the relatively brief evaluation of the physical demands (Figure 3).

7

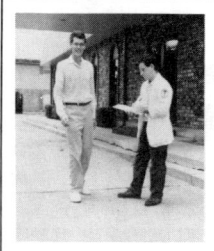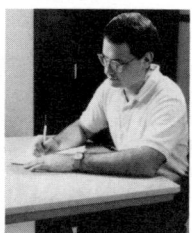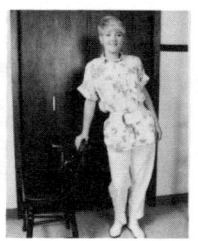

Figure 3

The objectivity of the tests comes from three sources. First, the individual performs a specific activity that tests the given physical demand. For example, the subtest for running is "run a distance of 30 yards on a level surface, turning at least once." (Figure 4)

Second, there are cross-assessments of the physical demands within the subtests. For example, the stooping subtest crosses with both that of unilateral lifting and reaching in the low plane. A patient who is fully aware that he or she is bending from the waist or stooping repeatedly when performing the stooping subtest may feign in the ability to stoop. If the patient automatically stoops when reaching in the low plane or when performing the subtest of one-handed lifting, he or she will provide the cross assessment for stooping. If the patient is unable to forward flex sufficiently to reach the low plane while being tested for stooping, but stoops to reach the low plane when lifting, the therapist becomes suspicious (Figure 5).

Finally, there should be a correlation between the symptoms expected from the person's medical condition and the functional limitations actually exhibited in performance of the tests. However, if the diagnosis is not fully established and the SPCE is being used to assist in the diagnosis, or if the therapist notes inconsistent behavior that may indicate a magnification of symptoms (Matheson 1984) or a secondary medical problem, any lack of correlation is of significance in the overall rehabilitation plan for the patient.

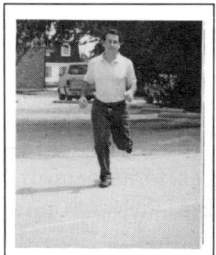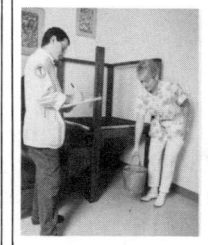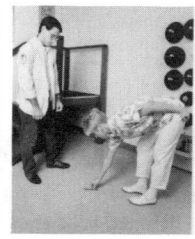

Figure 4   **Figure 5**

RATINGS

Ratings of the SPCE are based on the normal human developmental scale. Because the test is designed for persons of working age (16 to 70 years old), all persons within this age range have the potential to perform all 20 physical demands. However, the levels of endurance, agility, and spontaneity of movement are primary developmental factors that diminish with age. Thus, older persons may not be able to safely perform the physical tasks requiring high levels of agility, balance, and freedom of movement (for example, jumping and running). Since the patient is measured against a cross section of able bodied persons of the same age range and sex, limited ability in the older age range does not necessarily denote functional disability.

Various aspects of the patient's performance are rated during performance of each subtest. Among these are endurance, ability, and safety. Each aspect is given one of four ratings: within normal range, fair, poor, or unable (to perform). If for some reason the subtest is not administered, "not tested" is indicated. "Within normal range" denotes performance within the normal range for a person of the same sex and age range as the patient being tested. "Fair" denotes a performance somewhat less than within the normal range, and "poor" refers to a substantially less than normal performance. If the patient is unable to accomplish the activity called for, the performance is rated "unable." The designation of plus or minus may be used to indicate the upper or lower end of any of the rating ranges. Established norms or guidelines of norms, when available, should be used. Established norms are currently available for grasp strength (Mathiowetz et al. 1985), walking (Snook, 1978), and lifting.

A short section for comments is provided with each subtest evaluating physical demands to explain any ratings that fall short of the normal range in the performance of the test. Comments should be brief and concise explanations of the deficit in function and nothing more.

EQUIPMENT

The equipment needed to administer the SPCE is durable, inexpensive, and readily available for purchase or easily fabricated. Equipment that must be fabricated (or purchased through a specialty vendor) includes stairs, ramps, boxes, weighted cans, and sandbag weights (Figure 6) (See equipment list, Figure 12). Other equipment, such as ladders, pails, wheelbarrows, and blocks and tackles may be purchased from a local hardware store or marine supply

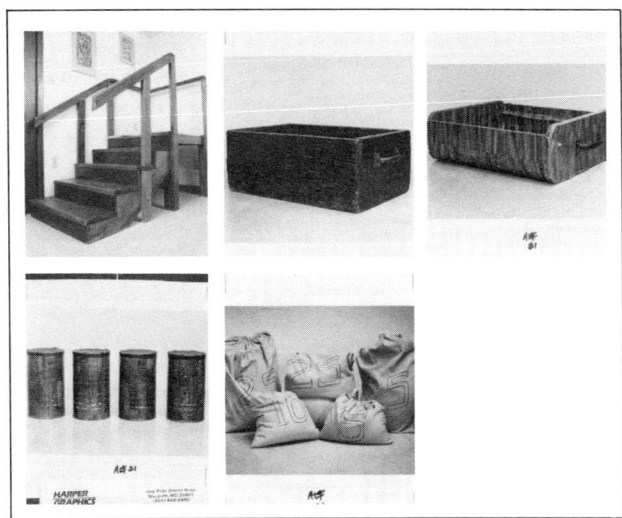

Figure 6

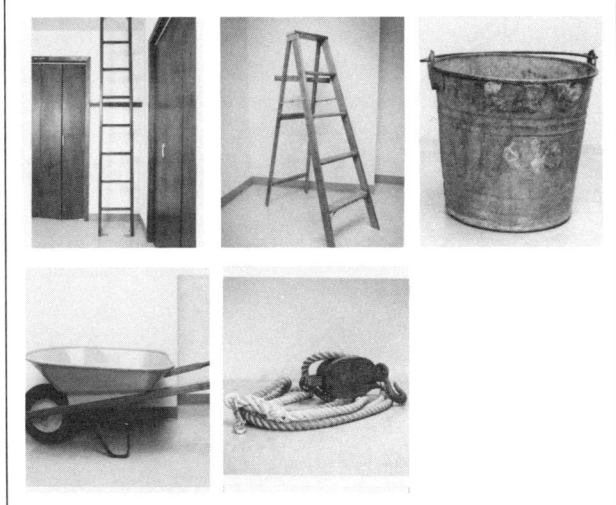

Figure 7

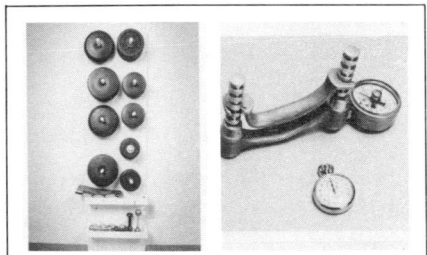

Figure 8

store (Figure 7). Disk and cuff weights, a stop watch, and a Jamar dynamometer may be purchased from a rehabilitation equipment company (Figure 8).

The available budget may determine the quality of the equipment. With an ample budget, hardwoods, rather than plywood or pine, may be selected to build stairs, ramp, and boxes, or they may be purchased commercially (Figure 9). The low budget facility may choose to build the equipment out of common types of woods. The price of stop watches, wheelbarrows, and ladders also varies. Items such as stop watch, disk and cuff weights, and Jamar dynamometer may already be available to the therapist in the occupational therapy department.

SPACE

As with equipment, space needed to administer the SPCE may be minimal or ample, depending upon what is available. Those with limited space may need to consider the use of multipurpose or public space. For instance, for the walking subtest, a hallway or sidewalk might be used as a straight walkway of 15 yards or more before turning. This is preferable to walking in a room where multiple turns would be necessary.

Stairs and boxes are used for multiple subtests, thereby contributing to space efficiency. Also, equipment may be stored in a space-saving manner. Therefore, if one must operate within limited space, the SPCE can be tailored to fit economically. Floor space as small as 200 square feet can be adequate for storage and administration of the SPCE, with some access to public or multipurpose space.

ADMINISTRATION

The SPCE is designed to be administered by occupational therapists, whose unique professional background and knowledge of normal growth and development, kinesiology, activity analysis, the behavioral sciences, and medical conditions help them to make accurate ratings.

Physical therapists with special interests and training are also able to administer and rate the SPCE accurately. Special training is needed because physical therapists assess one's physical capabilities largely from a clinical standpoint, whereas occupational therapists make an assessment from a clinical and functional standpoint. The training serves to expand the physical therapist's approach to assessment. A collaborative team of occupational and physical therapists can be very effective in the administration of the SPCE.

Most important is the need for the therapist to establish and maintain rapport with the patient. The language the therapist uses to instruct the patient in each subtest is not standardized. Rather, it is at the discretion of the therapist to use language the patient understands in order to promote maximum performance and a feeling of ease. The therapist should

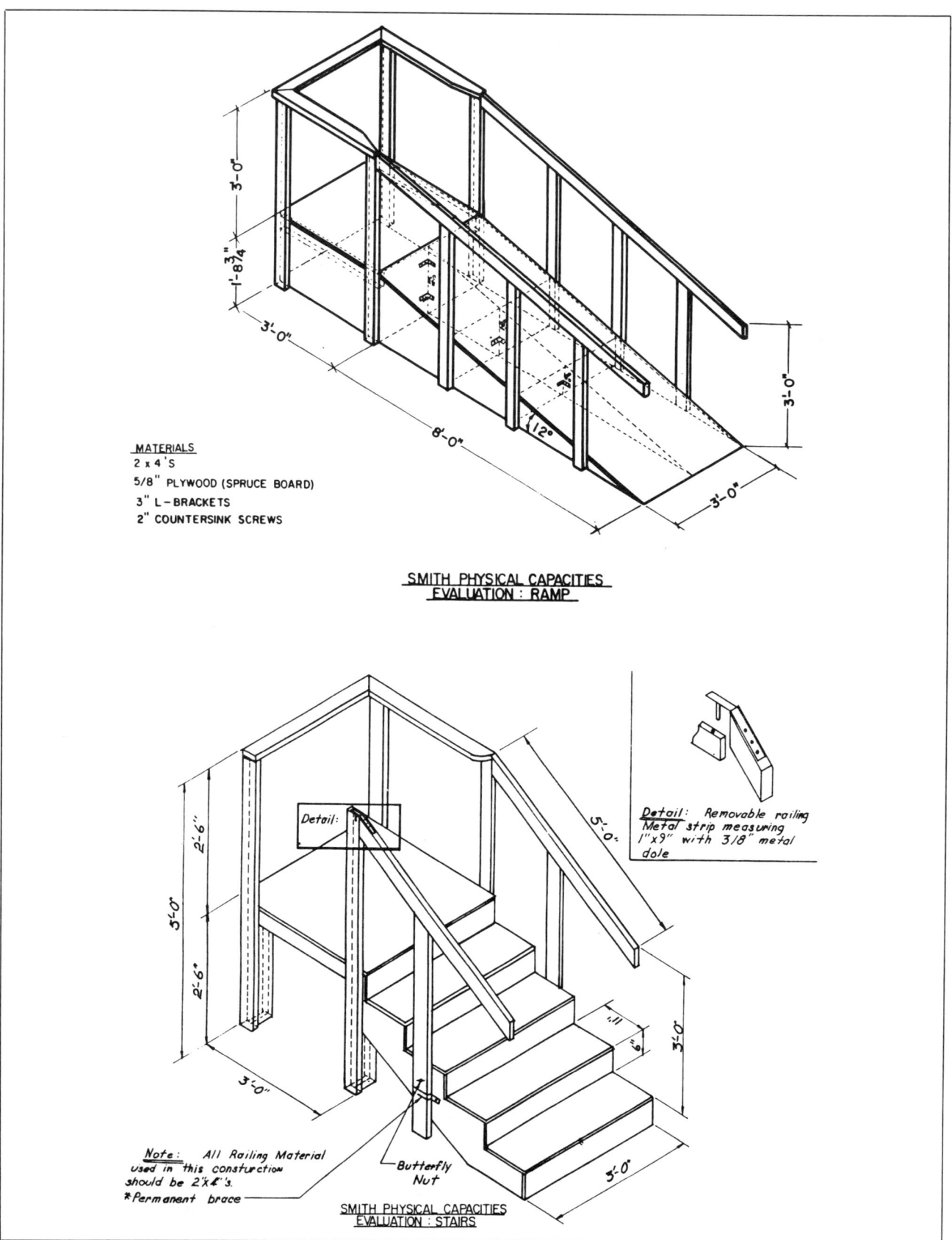

MATERIALS
2 x 4 'S
5/8" PLYWOOD (SPRUCE BOARD)
3" L – BRACKETS
2" COUNTERSINK SCREWS

SMITH PHYSICAL CAPACITIES
EVALUATION : RAMP

Detail: Removable railing
Metal strip measuring
1"x9" with 3/8" metal
dole

Note: All Railing Material
used in this consturction
should be 2"x4"'s.
*Permanent brace

Butterfly
Nut

SMITH PHYSICAL CAPACITIES
EVALUATION : STAIRS

Figure 9

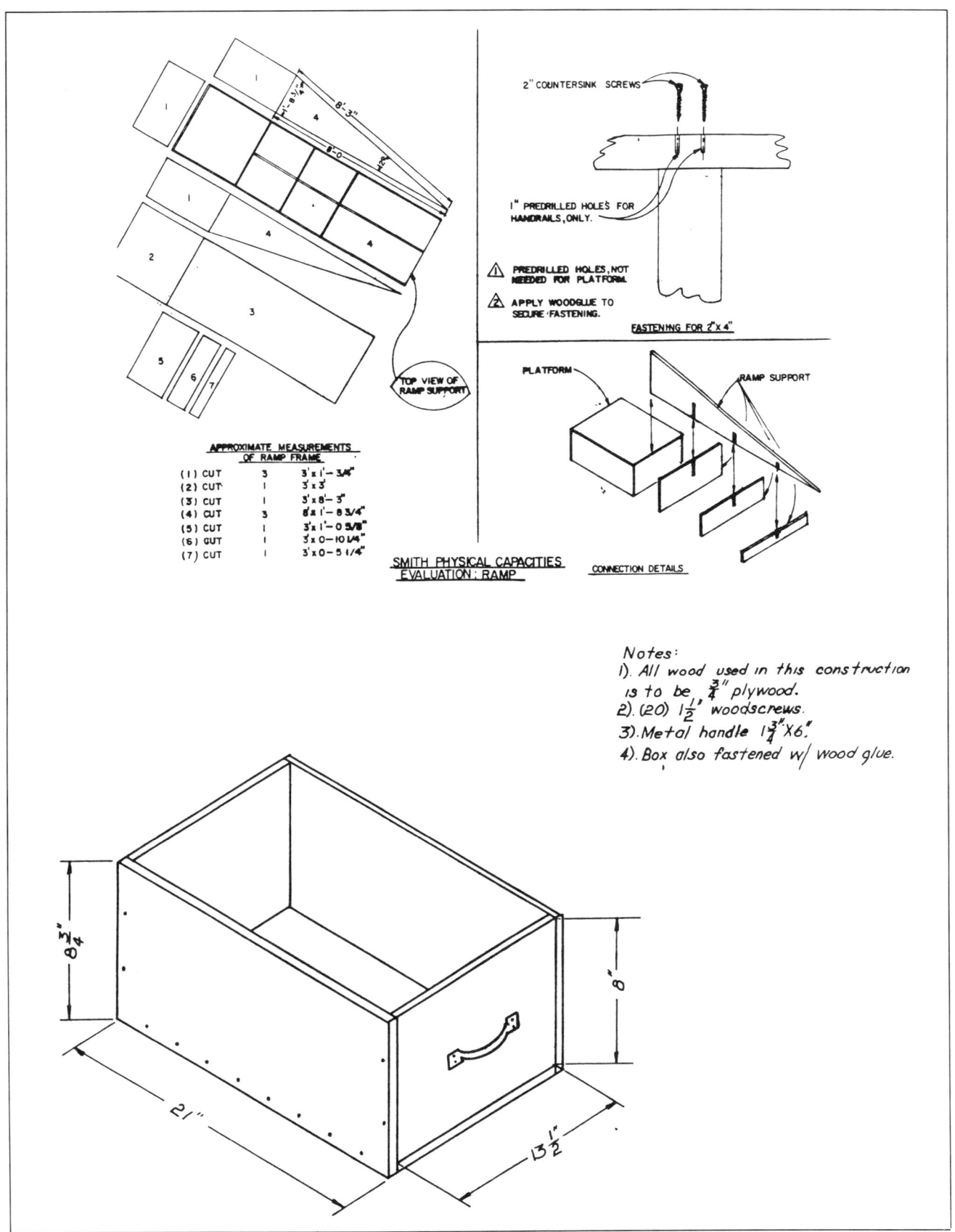

Figure 9 *Continued*

use a positive approach to assist the patient's best effort. The malingerer will be identified through inconsistent performance when the test is interpreted.

During the administration of each subtest, the therapist should be diligent in documenting compensatory biomechanical substitutions used in the individual's performance. Abnormal physiological responses (e.g., feeling lightheaded, blanching, flushing, and perspiring) should be noted, and emotional reactions (e.g., depression, anxiety, and agitation) should be monitored.

As in any evaluation, the therapist's professional judgment must be used in determining whether it is safe for the patient to continue to engage in the physical demands of a subtest. Any observation of physical or emotional discomfort or fatigue is recorded, and endurance, physiological responses, balance, and judgment all enter into the evaluation, along with medical precautions.

A positive approach by the therapist in administering the SPCE cannot be overemphasized. Frequently, a person who has suffered major physical trauma and subsequent long or multiple hospitalizations and discomfort will be unable to perform optimally without a supportive and positive therapist. The same holds true for the person who is depressed, has low self-esteem, or is fearful of attempting activities.

INTERPRETATION

In interpreting the SPCE, the therapist is readily able to identify the physical demands that the patient is able to execute in a normal or abnormal fashion (impaired, severely impaired, or absent). These can then be compared with the physical demands of the patient's job. During the testing, the therapist may have discussed with the patient each of the physical demands as they were tested in order to determine whether they were required in the patient's customary job. The responses can then be corroborated further by researching the specific job and its physical demands in the *Dictionary of Occupational Titles* (U.S. Dept. of Labor, 1991). This publication provides comprehensive information about all known jobs in the national labor market.

Since there is a subtest for 20 physical demands, comparisons may be easily made. The specified physical demands are considered primary to the particular job. Therefore, the therapist may also wish to consider any secondary or unique requirements discussed with the patient. It may even be of benefit to explore the patient's ability to perform the non-job-related physical demands of daily life: family and home responsibilities, leisure and avocational interests, and self-maintenance. A structured interview

may be administered (Figure 10). Once the patient's physical capacities are determined, further intervention in various forms—surgical, medical, psychological, physical, rehabilitation, vocational rehabilitation, vocational placement, and legal testimony—may be considered.

The format of the SPCE report is determined by the therapist's purpose in using and communicating the results. Formats may range from brief and graphic to detailed and descriptive. The standardized SPCE is formatted so that it can stand alone as a report, be incorporated into a narrative report as a specific reference, or be attached to a brief narrative summary. When a full functional evaluation is done for legal, industrial, or rehabilitation purposes, the completed standardized form is usually included in the report. However, when the purpose of the evaluation is to establish a data base for treatment planning and the document will be used only intradepartmentally, the standardized form itself is sufficient, supplemented by an evaluation note in the patient's record.

A summary of findings may be reported in profile form, which may be a desirable means of monitoring progress when successive progress evaluations are required. A profile form may be presented in a graphic format as a quick reference for the vocational evaluator to learn the parameters of physical capacities used in matching a client to the physical demands of a job (Figure 11).

The SPCE standardized form is designed for adding data simply by keeping the form on a word processor. If word processor capabilities are not available, data may be typed in the appropriate spaces (Figure 12). A SPCE Administrator's Guide Rating and Standards precedes the SPCE form.

It is the responsibility of the therapist to report the findings and his or her opinion of the patient's physical capacities in the most meaningful and time-efficient manner for the specific purpose of the testing. The report should include subjective and objective data that can be compared sequentially.

THE FUNCTIONAL EVALUATION INCORPORATING THE SPCE

The SPCE is valuable for assessing overall physical capabilities when baseline data are needed for planning an individual's rehabilitation program. The SPCE is also useful for defining a person's level of physical capacities, which is often required by the vocational evaluator, employer, or attorney seeking information to assess whether a person is able to meet the physical demands of usual work or future work placement. The functional evaluation incorporates the SPCE into its framework and examines three areas identified in Reed's and Sanderson's (1980) *Theory of Competence and Adaptations*: self-maintenance, work, and play. Besides the SPCE performance component, two other well-defined components of the functional evaluation are the review of medical documentation and the activity interview.

Review of Medical Documentation

Methods of gathering medical information are those commonly employed by occupational therapists. The patient's medical report, the primary source of information, is frequently supplemented by information presented at team treatment conferences, by direct discussion with the physician, and by communication with the patient during the SPCE. Medical documentation should indicate those medical factors directly affecting the testing and performance and should include the physician's assessment of the patient's prognosis and plans for surgical and medical intervention. Information should also be provided about medical contraindications, especially for activity, and precautions.

If the evaluation is solely for legal purposes, the therapist may not have direct access to medical information prior to the evaluation. In these cases, if an attorney is the referral source, copies of pertinent medical reports should be requested by the therapist prior to seeing the patient. If the patient is self-referred, the therapist may wish to obtain a release from the patient to obtain records from the doctor. Alternatively, the patient may possess his or her own medical records which the therapist may, with permission, copy.

It is not unusual for the therapist to become aware of additional health problems or medical impairments as the evaluation progresses. Hearing loss, a visual problem, or a residual physical deficit from an old injury or illness are among the most common discoveries.

Activity Interview

A review of the patient's pre- and post-injury activities encompasses activities in all spheres of the person's life and gives the therapist an idea of the patient's usual activity level, transferable skills, and knowledge.

If the information is gathered through a single interview, the interview skills of the therapist aid in quickly establishing rapport to obtain a thorough and complete picture of the activity level in the person's life. If the patient is being treated over a period of time, the therapist may choose to do a basic initial evaluation and then continue to gather details from discussion during treatment sessions. Sequential in-

terviewing sessions may enable the patient to feel more comfortable. Conversely, sequential interviewing may give the patient time to consider imagined or real problems particularly if he or she has tendencies toward symptom magnification. These problems may then influence the report.

The purpose of the functional evaluation will determine the steps of the activity interview. For instance, if the focus is on determining the patient's capacity to work, then discussion of leisure activities or family and home responsibilities may be eliminated and topics of education and personal care may be merely touched upon. Conversely, if the evaluation is for legal purposes, the therapist will undoubtedly wish to complete an in-depth interview. Following are several of the many possible topics that are covered in the activity interview.

Educational Background

In exploring the educational background of the patient, all educational and training experiences need to be discussed. Commonly, these experiences may include one or more of the following:

1. Formal elementary and secondary education
2. Postsecondary education
3. Postgraduate studies, including doctoral studies
4. Vocational/technical or business school courses
5. Specialized vocational school courses
6. Training under governmental programs, such as the Comprehensive Employment Training Act (CETA), Job Corps, Manpower Training Act
7. Military school courses
8. Work related continuing education
9. Adult enrichment education courses, such as flower arranging, sailing, and the study of a foreign language
10. Self-study achievement (e.g., general education diploma)
11. Social, physical, or emotional rehabilitation training.

With an understanding of the patient's interest in and ability to profit from educational endeavors, the therapist is able to advise the patient regarding the potential for a career redetermination through the use of transferable skills. If a person has a language barrier, a low educational level, a head injury, or a brain trauma, the therapist should explore his or her basic literacy. Responses to simple questions regarding the ability to read the newspaper, write one's name and address, count personal change, tell time, and read a ruler will serve as a cursory determination for illiteracy, functional illiteracy, or literacy.

Persons with visual, auditory, speech, and dominant hand problems may have problems using their knowledge. Those who have limited or no knowledge of English are handicapped educationally. However, fluency in another language may be an advantageous work skill.

The educational background portion of the activity interview allows the therapist to identify a possible learning disability, deficient I.Q., or psychological condition. Through discussion, it may be learned that the person had been placed in a special education class in school, or repeated one or more grades.

Work History

Since a detailed account of the patient's activity level is the focus of the interview, it is not essential to have a complete work history. Specific employers, detailed dates of employment, and an account of all jobs ever held are of little significance. Rather, the emphasis is on examining the various types of work done, the major changes in occupation or profession that may have occurred, and the dedication the person has had to work and career.

Primary jobs as well as secondary and avocational jobs should be discussed. Some individuals may have held two jobs simultaneously, such as that of car parking attendant during the day and an office building porter at night. Others may have held side jobs to supplement their income and provide relaxation in off-hours, such as a registered nurse who teaches a dance class once a week; or a tugboat captain who does auto mechanics for friends when off-duty.

For those who have been in the military, a knowledge of their military work assignments is helpful. Their activities during their tour of duty may transfer to civilian life. Also, people having served prison terms usually have held work assignments while in prison, and these are useful to know.

The work history portion of the activity interview sheds light on the patient's skills and knowledge acquired through working. It also reveals a preference for outdoor or indoor work, and it indicates whether the individual's personality is best suited to dealing with people, objects, or data.

Family and Home Responsibilities

Family and home responsibilities may vary from minor (e.g., the single apartment dweller) to extensive (e.g., the rural farmer). Of particular interest are the responsibilities established prior to illness or injury and how the person is coping to meet these responsibilities. Responsibilities may include yard and home maintenance; household activities such as cooking, shopping, laundry, and cleaning; child care;

the care of barnyard animals or pets; auto maintenance; and gardening. Frequently, people will have additional responsibilities outside their immediate home. For instance, cutting grass or shoveling snow for parents and taking a mother for weekly grocery shopping are not uncommon responsibilities. Information on the level of responsibilities established prior to illness or injury and how the person is coping to meet these at the present time is important.

Information on family and home responsibilities gives the therapist an idea of the patient's ability to carry out the activities of daily life. Those who have been unable to return to the usual level of activity may be placing a hardship on other family members, or may be suffering marital discord. This in turn may be causing the patient's stress.

Leisure-time Interests

Leisure activities, including recreational, social, and religious activities as well as other means of relaxation and self-fulfillment, may be family, civic, or group oriented, and may be partaken as part of a group or individually. It is not uncommon for the patient to need some assistance in identifying these interests. Consequently, the therapist may need to ask questions, for example, "Do you enjoy fishing . . . reading . . . working on your car?" or "Is there anything you do through your church?"

It is important to determine whether, and if so, why, usual interests have changed or been modified. If the patient has begun to develop new leisure-time interests in accordance with the physical capacities, the therapist must know. A restriction of involvement in leisure activities may result in social isolation or even family problems.

Personal Care Capabilities

The therapist must assess the patient's ability to get ready for work, as well as manage transportation to and from work. Among the areas to be touched on in this part of the interview are the ability to manage feeding, dressing, bathing, grooming, and transportation. The latter may be driving, taking public buses, car pooling, taking commuter trains, planes, helicopters, or subways, or riding a motorcycle or bicycle. If the patient is not independent in personal care, it is important to know who is providing assistance and whether the situation is acceptable. It is also important to know how the dependent person manages travel, and whether travel is only for occasional appointments or necessary for leisure, daily life, and work activities.

Age

It is important to know the birth date of the patient; if a redetermination of a career is necessary, age is an important consideration (Figure 13).

Summary

The Functional Evaluation, using the SPCE as the performance component, is useful in establishing the patient's current level of functioning and identifying disability in each area of the person's life including self-maintenance, work and play. While the therapist administers the SPCE to all patients, components of the functional evaluation are administered in certain areas to gather specific details on the patient's activity level in one or more specific areas. The therapist may focus on specific areas of activity depending upon the purpose of the SPCE.

REFERENCES

Matheson, L. *Symptom Magnification: Clinical Strategies for Identification of Malingering* (audiotape). Torrance, CA: Discovery House, 1984.

Mathiowetz, V., Kashman, N., Volland, G., Weber, K., Dowe, M., and Rogers,S. "Grip and Pinch Strength Normative Data for Adults." *Archives of Physical Medicine and Rehabilitation* 66 (February 1985): pp. 69-74.

Mathiowetz, V., Wiemer, D., and Federman, S. "Grip and Pinch Strength: Norms for Six- to Nineteen- Year Olds." *American Journal of Occupational Therapy* 40, (1986): pp. 705-11.

Reed, K.L. and Sanderson, S.R. *Concepts of Occupational Therapy.* Baltimore: Williams and Wilkins, 1980.

Snook, S. "The Design of Manual Handling Tasks." *Ergonomics* 21, (1978): (12) 963-985.

U.S. Dept. of Labor. *Dictionary of Occupational Titles.* Washington, DC: U.S. Government Printing Office, 1977.

U.S. Dept of Labor. *Selected Characteristics of Occupations Defined in the Dictionary of Occupational Titles.* Washington, DC: U.S. Government Printing Office, 1981.

GUIDE FOR INTERVIEWING CLIENTS IN CONJUNCTION

WITH A FUNCTIONAL EVALUATION

INTRODUCTION:

The following topics should be covered in an in-depth interview prior to administering a Physical Capacities Evaluation or other specific evaluations in determining one's functional capacities.

TOPICS:

1. Work history

   A. As complete a work history as possible should be obtained from the client.

   B. The exact dates of employment and company names are of little importance.

   C. Of importance are approximate durations which a job was held and at what time in the client's career life he was engaged in this work, as well as the job classification and duties.

   D. Military Duty

      a. Specific assignments while in the military.

2. Education:

   A. The highest grade which the client obtained.

   B. Any education beyond high school; specialized or general

   C. Any vocational education
      a. Include any short courses given specifically to train a person for their job, i.e. a two week course to operate a certain kind of machine.

      b. Any military "schools" which the client went to while in the military

Figure 10

      c. Any plans to return to school to up-grade either their education or vocational competence

      d. Any plans to involve themselves with Vocational Rehabilitation Services

3. Family and home responsibilities:

    A. Is the client married or single, divorced or separated

    B. Number of children client has and what actual contact and responsibilities he has to the children as well as any limitations he has in caring for the children.

    C. Does the client live in an apartment or a home.
      a. If in a home, is he responsible for yard and home maintenance.

      b. Does he take responsibility for his own car maintenance and/or repair.

      c. What responsibilities do other members of the household assume

      d. In all these areas, has there been any change since the client has become ill or injured.

    D. Does the client have a flower or vegetable garden.

    E. Does the client have any farm animals or animals which require significant care, i.e. tropical fish

4. Leisure time interests:

    A. This includes recreational, sport, religious, fraternal, social, and individual and/or hobby interests.

      a. Note where these may be particularly family oriented interests.

    B. This is usually the most difficult area for the client to relate as he does not think of leisure time activities as such. Therefore, you will probably need to give suggestions and do some probing in this area.

5. Driving:

    A. Does the client have a current driver's license and drive a car.

    B. Does the car have an automatic transmission, power brakes, and steering, or is it a standard transmission.

    C. Does the client have any other vehicles which he uses, i.e. pick-up truck or motorcycle, or bicycle

6. Personal care:

    A. Is the client able to accomplish his personal care independently

7. Date of birth

Figure 10 *Continued*

The Pain and Rehabilitation Center
● 3525 Prytania St. Suite 318 ● New Orleans, LA 70115 ● (504)899-5284 ●

SMITH PHYSICAL CAPACITIES EVALUATION SUMMARY PROFILE

Client's Name:_____ Birth Date:_____

Client's Occupation:_____

Therapist's Name:_____ Evaluation Date:_____

Medical Contra-indications:_____

_____

PHYSICAL DEMANDS OF CLIENT'S JOB COMPARED TO HIS PERFORMANCE OF THEM:

Reference: Dictionary of Occupational Titles, and Selected Characteristics
of Jobs Identified in the Dictionary of Occupational Titles (D.O.T.)

Evaluation Performance   Job Requirements

LIFT: Amt.____ Able____ Impaired____ Unable____ Job Rq.____ Amt.____

CARRY: Amt.____ Able____ Impaired____ Unable____ Job Rq.____ Amt.____

PUSH: Amt.____ Able____ Impaired____ Unable____ Job Rq.____ Amt.____

PULL: Amt.____ Able____ Impaired____ Unable____ Job Rq.____ Amt.____

BALANCE: Able____ Impaired____ Unable____ Job Rq.____

CLIMB: Able____ Impaired____ Unable____ Job Rq.____

STOOP: Able____ Impaired____ Unable____ Job Rq.____

KNEEL: Able____ Impaired____ Unable____ Job Rq.____

CROUCH: Able____ Impaired____ Unable____ Job Rq.____

CRAWL: Able____ Impaired____ Unable____ Job Rq.____

RUN: Able____ Impaired____ Unable____ Job Rq.____

JUMP: Able____ Impaired____ Unable____ Job Rq.____

SEE/HEAR: Able____ Impaired____ Unable____ Job Rq.____

RECLINE: Able____ Impaired____ Unable____ Job Rq.____

TALK: Able____ Impaired____ Unable____ Job Rq.____

GRASP: Able____ Impaired____ Unable____ Job Rq.____

REACH: Able____ Impaired____ Unable____ Job Rq.____

SIT: Able____ Impaired____ Unable____ Job Rq.____

STAND: Able____ Impaired____ Unable____ Job Rq.____

Client is able to ____ unable to ____ meet the physical demands of his job.

Client is able to meet the physical demands of: Sedentary ___ Light ___
     Medium ___ Heavy ___ Very Heavy ___ work as classified by the D.O.T.

Client is unable to meet the physical demands of competitive work:____

Figure 11

Professional Occupational Therapy Services, Inc.
2727 Houma Bouevard
Metairie, Louisiana 70006   Name: _____

                                             Date: _____

SMITH PHYSICAL CAPACITIES EVALUATION

This evaluation is designed to measure the gross functional capacities and limitations of a person. It is based upon the 20 broad physical demands which the U. S. Department of Labor utilizes in specifying the primary requisite physical demands for jobs in the national competitive labor market.

The evaluation is rated using the following rating scale. The standard of measure being a cross-section of persons of the same age range and sex as the person being evaluated.

Within Normal Range (WNR); Fair; Poor; Unable

Walking:
    Request:
    1.   To walk normally 100 yards on level surface, turning to reverse direction at least one (1) time.

    Performance:
            a.   Type of gait:
            b.   Appliances used:
            c.   Endurance:
            d.   Safety:
            e.   Ability to turn:

    2.   The client's estimate of distance and length of time they are able to walk.

    Estimate:
            a.   Distance inside:
            b.   Distance outside:
            c.   Time inside:
           ·d.   Time outside:

COMMENT: _____

_____

_____

_____

_____

_____

_____

_____

Figure 12

```
SMITH PHYSICAL CAPACITIES
EVALUATION - Page 2                    Name: _____

                                       Date: _____
```

Running:
    Request: To run 30 yards on a level surface turning to reverse direction at least one (1) time.

    Performance:
        a.   Ability:
        b.   Endurance:
        c.   Type of gait:
        d.   Safety:

    COMMENT: _____

_____

_____

_____

Jumping:
    Request: To jump from an 18", and then a 30" high platform onto level surface, landing on both feet.

    Performance:
        a.   Ability: 18": _____   30": _____
        b.   Balance: 18": _____   30": _____
        c.   Safety: 18": _____   30": _____
        d.   Endurance: 18": _____   30": _____

    COMMENT: _____

_____

_____

_____

Figure 12 *Continued*

```
SMITH PHYSICAL CAPACITIES
EVALUATION - Page 3                        Name: _____

                                           Date: _____



Climbing:
    Request:
    1.   Ramp (8' x 12°):   To walk up and down five (5) consecu-
         tive times.

    Performance:
         a.     Gait:
         b.     Endurance:
         c.     Use of appliances:

    2.   Stairs (5 steps, 6" rise, wooden tread):   To walk up
         and down two (2) times.

    Performance:
         a.     Safety:
         b.     Endurance:
         c.     Speed:
         d.     Use of handrail:
         e.     Use of appliances:
         f.     Foot-over-foot:
                Foot-by-foot:

    3.   Curbs (6", 12" and 18" high):
         To ascend and descend curbs once.

    Performance:
         a.     Ability:
                6":
                12":
                18":
         b.     Safety:
                6":
                12":
                18":
         c.     Appliances used:
                6":
                12":
                18":
         d.     Use of handrail:
                6":
                12":
                18":
```

Figure 12 *Continued*

```
SMITH PHYSICAL CAPACITIES
EVALUATION - Page 4                    Name: _____

                                       Date: _____
```

4. Straight Ladder (8', 11" rise):
    To climb up and down five (5) consecutive times.

    Performance:
    a. Foot-over-foot:
        Foot-by-foot:
    b. Hand-over-hand:
        Hand-on-rail:
        Hand-by-hand:
    c. Balance:
    d. Safety:
    e. Endurance:
    f. Ability:

5. Step Ladder (5, 12" rise): To climb up and down once
    carrying a 10 pound pail in the hand of client's
    choice.

    Performance:
    a. Foot-over-foot:
        Foot-by-foot:
    b. Balance:
    c. Safety:
    d. Endurance:

COMMENT: _____

_____

_____

_____

_____

_____

_____

_____

_____

_____

_____

Figure 12 *Continued*

```
SMITH PHYSICAL CAPACITIES
EVALUATION - Page 5                    Name: _____

                                       Date: _____




Crouching:
     Request: To work in a squatted position for three (3)
          minutes, alternately placing two pound cans (4" x8")
          from the floor to a 12" high shelf.

     Performance:
          a.    Ability to assume position:
          b.    Ability to carry out task:
          c.    Ability to regain standing'
          d.    Balance:
          e.    Endurance:


     COMMENT: _____

     _____

     _____

     _____

     _____

     _____


Lifting:
     Request:
     1.   Right Hand:  To alternately lift maximum weights in a
          pail from a waist-high surface to floor and back five
          (5) consecutive times.

     Performance:
          a.    Number of pounds:
          b.    Ability:
          c.    Balance:
          d:    Endurance:
          e.    Ability to grasp:

     2.   Left Hand:  To repeat (1) using the left hand.

     Performance:
          a.    Number of pounds:
          b.    Ability:
          c.    Balance:
          d.    Endurance:
          e.    Ability to grasp:
```

Figure 12 *Continued*

```
SMITH PHYSICAL CAPACITIES
EVALUATION - Page 6                    Name: _____

                                       Date: _____
```

3. Both Hands: To alternately lift maximum weight in a box from a waist-high surface to floor five (5) consecutive times.

    Performance:
    a. Number of pounds:
    b. Ability:
    c. Balance:
    d. Endurance:
    e. Ability to grasp: Right: Left:

    COMMENT: _____

    _____

    _____

    _____

    _____

    _____

    _____

    _____

Carrying:
    Request: To bimanually carry the maximum weight in a box 25 yards, while walking on a level surface. The box taken from, and returned to, a waist-high surface.

    Performance:
    a. Number of pounds:
    b. Ability:
    c. Balance:
    d. Endurance:
    e. Type of gait:
    f. Ability to grasp: Right: Left:

    COMMENT: _____

    _____

    _____

    _____

Figure 12 *Continued*

SMITH PHYSICAL CAPACITIES
EVALUATION - Page 7

Name: _____

Date: _____

Pushing: Push-Pull:
    Request:
    1.   To push a wheelbarrow (heavy duty with inflated rubber tire) for 25 yards on a level surface with the maximum load client able to handle.

    Performance:
        a.   Ability:
        b.   Balance on turning:
        c.   Endurance:
        d.   Number of pounds:
              Number of pounds at handles:

    2.   To alternately push and pull bimanually, to arm's length, the maximum in a weighted box on a waist-high rough surface, 10 times, first from a standing and then a sitting position.

    Performance: a.   Number of Pounds: Standing: Sitting:
                b.   Ability: Standing: Sitting:
                c.   Endurance: Standing: Sitting:
                d.   Range of Motion: Back: Arms:
                e.   Ability to grasp: Right: Left:

COMMENT: _____

_____

_____

_____

_____

_____

Pulling:
    Request: To alternately pull and lower, in a hand-over-hand fashion the maximum weight on a single pulley (3/4" cotton rope) 10 consecutive times.

    Performance:
        a.   Number of pounds:
        b.   Ability:
        c.   Balance:
        d.   Endurance:
        e.   Reach:
        f.   Visual Monitoring:
        g.   Ability to grasp:
                Right:
                Left:

Figure 12 *Continued*

```
SMITH PHYSICAL CAPACITIES
EVALUATION  - Page 8                    Name: _____

                                        Date: _____



        COMMENT:  _____

_____

_____

_____
```

Stooping:
    Request: To perform for three minutes, alternately standing
    and stooping, while bimanually placing 2 lb. cans (4" x 8")
    on a 42" high shelf to the floor.

    Performance:
        a.   Ability:
        b.   Endurance:
        c.   Ability to grasp:
                  Right:
                  Left:

```
        COMMENT:  _____

_____

_____

_____
```

Reaching:
    Request:
    1.   Overhead: From a standing position to:
        a.   Bimanually pick-up a 10 lb. box from a waist-high
              surface, place it on an imaginary overhead shelf,
              and then return it to the waist-high surface, one
              (1) time.

        b.   To reach a pencil, first with right and then with
              left hand, at the extreme of reach at right, left
              and across body; and at the midline, then to reach
              bimanually directly in front of the body.

    Performance: a.   Ability: 10 lbs.:
                                 Small Object:
                  b.   Range of Motion: Right: Left:
                                         Back: Neck:
                  c.   Balance:
                  d.   Coordination:
                  e.   Grasp: Right: Left:
                  f.   Endurance:

Figure 12 *Continued*

SMITH PHYSICAL CAPACITIES
EVALUATION - Page 9

Name: _____

Date: _____

2. <u>Immediate</u>:
   a. From a standing position to bimanually reach forward and pick-up a 10 lb. box from a waist-high surface and return it to that surface.

   b. Repeat 1.b. in the immediate plane with therapist holding the pencil at the various points of reach. The client is seated in a straight chair.

Performance: a. Ability: 10 lbs.:   Small Obj.:
             b. Range of Motion: Right: Left:
                                 Back: Neck:
             c. Balance:
             d. Coordination:
             e. Grasp: Right: Left:
             f. Endurance:

3. <u>Low</u>: <u>Sitting</u>:
   a. Repeat 1.b., the therapist placing the pencil on the floor, at designated points while the client sits in a straight chair, and reaches.

Performance: a. Ability:
             b. Range of Motion: Right: Left:
                                 Back: Neck:
             c. Balance:
             d: Coordination:
             e. Grasp: Right: Left:
             f. Endurance:

4. <u>Low</u>: <u>Standing</u>:
   a. Repeat 1.b. the therapist placing the pencil on the floor, at designated points, while the client stands in one position.

Performance: a. Ability:
             b. Range of Motion: Right: Left:
                                 Back: Neck:
             c. Balance:
             d. Coordination:
             e. Grasp: Right: Left:
             f. Endurance:

<u>COMMENT</u>: _____

_____

_____

_____

Figure 12 *Continued*

```
SMITH PHYSICAL CAPACITIES
EVALUATION - Page 10                    Name: _____

                                        Date: _____
```

_____

_____

_____

_____

```
Kneeling:
     Request:   To  assume  a  kneeling   position   on  the  floor,
          keeping  the  back straight, and maintain  the position
          for one minute.

     Performance:
          a.  Ability to assume position:
          b.  Ability to regain standing:
          c.  Balance:
          d.  Endurance:
          e.  Ability:
```

COMMENT: _____

_____

_____

_____

```
Crawling:
     Request:   To  crawl  on a level floor  eight  feet forward and
          then backward with head and shoulders low.

     Performance:
          a.  Type crawl:
                    4-point:
                    3-point:
                    Other:
          b.  Speed:
          c.  Ability:
          d.  Endurance:
```

COMMENT: _____

_____

_____

_____

Figure 12 *Continued*

```
SMITH PHYSICAL CAPACITIES
EVALUATION - Page 11                 Name:  _____

                                     Date:  _____


Reclining:
     Request:   To assume a  backlying position on the floor.  When
               in position  turn to one  side, then the other, and  then
               face-lying.  Return to standing position.

     Performance:
          a.    Ability to:
                    Assume Position:
                    Regain Standing:
                    Turn Right:
                    Turn Left:
                    Turn Face-lying:
          b.    Comfort on:
                    Right:
                    Left:
                    Face:
                    Back:


     COMMENT:  _____

     _____

     _____

     _____


Turning:
     Request:
     a.   With the  client standing  with their right side  to  a
          waist-high surface,  reach and lift  the maximum weight
          in  a   box from this surface by only turning the trunk.
          Place the box  on  the floor and then return it to waist-
          high surface only using rotation of the trunk.
     b.   Repeat, standing with client's  left side  to the waist
          high shelf.

     Performance:  a.  Ability to:      Right:          Left:
                   b.  Balance:         Right:          Left:
                   c.  Endurance:       Right:          Left:
                   d.  Number of pounds:


     Comment:  _____

     _____

     _____

     _____
```

Figure 12 *Continued*

```
SMITH PHYSICAL CAPACITIES
EVALUATION - Page 12                    Name: _____

                                        Date: _____


Balancing:
     Request:  To one-leg  stand, first  on the right and then the
          left leg, for 30 seconds each.

     Performance:  a.   Ability to
                        gain balance:    Right:          Left:
                   b.   Endurance:       Right:          Left:
                   c.   Leg Dominance:   Right:          Left:


     COMMENT: _____

     _____

     _____


Sitting:
     With what  ability is the  client able to get in and  out of a
     straight-back chair?  Client's estimate  of how long they can
     sit comfortably, and with what type of posture?

     Performance:
          a.   Ability to sit:
          b.   Ability to rise:
          c.   Estimated Time:
               Functional Posture:
               Non-Functional Posture:


     COMMENT: _____

     _____

     _____

     _____


Standing:
     What type   of  posture  and stance does the client exhibit?
     Client's estimate of time he can stand.

     Performance:
          a.   Posture:
          b.   Stance:
          c.   Estimate of Time:
               Functional Posture:
               Non-Functional Posture:
```

Figure 12 *Continued*

SMITH PHYSICAL CAPACITIES
EVALUATION - Page 13

Name: _____

Date: _____

COMMENT: _____

_____

_____

_____

_____

_____

Hand Grasp:
As measured with a dynamometer, the strength of the client's hand grasp.

Performance: a. Broad Grasp: Right: Left:
b. Tight Grasp: Right: Left:
c. Hand Dominance: Right: Left:

COMMENT: _____

_____

_____

Handling:
Therapist's estimate of the realistic maximum weight the client is able to handle comfortably. This includes lifting, carrying, pushing, and pulling. The estimate is based on the client's performance of these sub-tests.

a. Estimate:
b. Frequency: Routine: Frequent: Occasional:
c. Positions:
Overhead:
Frontal:
Right:
Left:
Low:

COMMENT: _____

_____

_____

_____

Figure 12 *Continued*

SMITH PHYSICAL CAPACITIES EVALUATION

EQUIPMENT LIST

CUSTOM BUILT: (See scale drawings)

1. Ramp with bilateral rails: 8' x 3' x 12
2. Stairs with landing and bilateral rails: 5 steps, 6" rises, wooden tread (one rail removable)
3. Wooden box with bilateral handles: 12" x 20" x 8"; 10 lbs.

CUSTOM FABRICATED:

4. Sandbags with loop closures: three 25 lb. bags, one 10 lb. bag, and two 5 lb. bags. (May be made of denim with awning cord drawstring closures. Bags should be double with the inner bag of sand made such as a beanbag. Sand may be purchased in a hardware store).
5. Wooden fruit lug box with bilateral handles: These boxes measure about $5\frac{1}{2}$" x $17\frac{1}{2}$" x 14" and weigh about $\frac{1}{2}$ lb. Supermarkets throw them out and may be picked up there at no charge. Screen door handles should be attached at both 14" ends. The box may be covered with contact paper to make more attractive.
6. Four (4) large juice cans (4" x 8"; 48 oz.) filled with 2 lbs. of sand and sealed. Optionally the cans may be covered with contact paper to make more attractive.

COMMERCIALLY AVAILABLE:

Available at Hardware Store:

7. One 10 quart galvanized pail.
8. One wooden straight ladder: 8' with 11" rises.
9. One folding step-ladder: 5' with 12" rises.
10. One heavy duty wheelbarrow with inflated rubber tire. And tire pump.

Available through Rehabilitation/Therapy Equipment Supplier:

11. One exercise mat at least 8' long. (Or may use carpeted area or piece of carpet).
12. One hundred or more pound disk weight set.
13. One each of the following cuff weights: $\frac{1}{2}$ lb., 1 lb., 2 lb., and 3 lb.
14. One stopwatch.
15. One Jamar hand dyanomometer (all stainless steel model)

Available at Boat Supply Store:

16. One large single pulley with 3/4" cotton rope (approximately 15') with snaphook attachment.

Available through Office Supply and Furniture Store:

17. Chairs: One straight backed chair with arms and one without arms. Suggested: a captain's and a mate's chair.
18. One ballpoint pen.

Miscellaneous:

19. Fastenings to securely fasten pulley to ceiling and straight ladder to ceiling and floor.

Figure 12 *Continued*

STAGES OF WORK CAREER LIFE

STAGE	AGE SPAN	TOTAL YEARS
<u>EARLY CAREER YEARS</u>		
Early, Early Career	16 – 29 Years	14
Mid, Early Career	16 – 20 Years	5
Late, Early Career	21 – 25 Years	5
	26 – 29 Years	4
<u>MID-CAREER YEARS</u>		
Early, Mid Career	30 – 55 Years	25
Mid, Mid Career	30 – 39 Years	10
Late, Mid Career	40 – 49 Years	10
	50 – 55 Years	5
<u>LATE CAREER YEARS</u>		
Early, Late Career	56 – 70 Years	15
Mid, Late Career	56 – 60 Years	5
Late, Late Career	51 – 65 Years	5
	66 – 70 Years	5

References: U.S. Department of Labor
Social Security Administration

Figure 13

32

CHAPTER THREE

THE BAXTER PHYSICAL CAPACITIES EVALUATION

THE BAXTER PHYSICAL CAPACITIES EVALUATION (BPCE) is administered to patients who have sustained upper extremity injuries or disease severe enough to cause the physician to question whether the patient's physical capacity is sufficient for performing his or her regular job. Each evaluation is designed to test the unique occupational requirements of each patient.

The majority of referrals from physicians are for evaluation of a patient's ability to return to a regular job. However, referrals from attorneys, insurance claims adjusters, and vocational rehabilitation counselors are made for defining the patient's physical ability to perform a specific classification of work as defined in the *Dictionary of Occupational Titles* (U.S. Dept. of Labor, 1991), so that vocational placement can proceed. The five levels of work are as follows:

Sedentary work (S): Lifting 10 lb. maximum and occasionally lifting and/or carrying such articles as dockets, ledgers, and small tools. Although a sedentary job is defined as one which involves sitting, a certain amount of walking and standing is often necessary in carrying out job duties. Jobs are sedentary if walking and standing are required only occasionally and other sedentary criteria are met.

Light Work (L): Lifting 20 lb. maximum with frequent lifting and/or carrying of objects weighing up to 10 lb. Even though the weight lifted may be only a negligible amount, a job is in this category when it requires walking or standing to a significant degree, or when it involves sitting most of the time with a degree of pushing and pulling of arm and/or leg controls.

Medium Work (M): Lifting 50 lb. maximum with frequent lifting and/or carrying of objects weighing up to 50 lb.

Heavy Work (H): Lifting 100 lb. maximum with frequent lifting and/or carrying of objects weighing up to 50 lb.

Very Heavy Work (V): Lifting objects in excess of 100 lb. with frequent lifting and/or carrying of objects weighing 50 lb. or more.

Also, referrals are accepted from attorneys and patients for documentation of physical abilities and restrictions related to all areas of occupational behavior, including self-maintenance, work, and play. The BPCE is used in the four models of practice: the rehabilitation model, the industrial model, the legal model, and the educational model.

TEST SELECTION

To plan for administration of the test, the therapist should clearly understand the purpose of the evaluation, so that all important areas of function are assessed. In addition, the therapist should review all the medical documentation and information about the individual's job. Several sources the therapist may use to collect data on the patient's job requirements include the *Dictionary of Occupational Titles* (U.S. Dept. of Labor 1991) job analyses, and on-site evaluations (see Chapter 5). The data collected supplies information that is used to plan each individual's BPCE.

The BPCE assesses four components of physical function. The biomechanical assessment reports on the patient's bony architecture, muscle and soft tissue status, and the presence of any amputations or limitations on joint motion. The sensory component assesses the patient's sensation in relation to hand-use ability for functional activity. The coordination component of the evaluation assesses the patient's speed and accuracy of hand use. Endurance is assessed as each patient's occupational activities require prolonged performance.

SELECTION OF BIOMECHANICAL TESTS

The therapist should administer tests that provide the most pertinent information regarding the patient's condition. For example, strength measurements are usually recorded with each patient, as a certain amount of strength is required in all work activities. Range-of-motion measurements are recorded with patients who present limitations. Patients with normal joint movement do not require measurement. Amputations of digits may simply be listed, whereas complete amputations of the hand may require a prosthetic check-out if a prosthesis is worn.

Manual muscle testing is performed when the patient's medical documentation indicates muscle weakness or peripheral nerve deficits. This type of test effectively isolates weakened muscles. Manual muscle testing can identify a muscle weakness when compensatory methods of lifting or carrying are indicated in the documentation. Specific biomechanical tests should be used when there are certain physical demands required in an individual's occupation. If the patient must reach, handle, and manipulate objects, the range of motion test, grip and pinch test, and coordination test should be performed. If the patient must lift, carry, and push objects, a grip test, a manual lifting test, and the Smith Physical Capacities Evaluation (SPCE) should be administered.

Individuals who have sustained fractures, crush injuries, joint injuries, amputations, and injuries of muscles or nerves should be assessed for biomechanical limitations. Based on the site and extent of the injury, the biomechanical function of the patient's hand or arm may be affected. For example, ankylosis of an individual's index proximal interphalangeal joint in partial flexion may not adversely affect the ability to manipulate small objects. However, a flexion contracture of the proximal interphalangeal joint of the small finger may adversely affect an individual's ability to handle tools. The patient may not be able to safely grasp and control tools for prolonged work sessions due to the joint contracture. The tests selected must correlate the patient's biomechanical measurements with both functional ability and restrictions.

SELECTION OF SENSORY COMPONENTS

The sensory component of the BPCE measures a patient's level of sensation and relates functional use to sensory function. If the physical demands of a patient's job require physical manipulation and feeling, the sensory component should be evaluated. Many patients have jobs that require the use of their hands around moving machinery or in extreme temperatures. During the data gathering process, patients should be questioned about the sensory function of their hands. However, it is important to objectively evaluate sensory function through the use of one or more sensory tests.

Many physicians are familiar with the administration of the two-point discrimination test. This quick and easy-to-administer test is suggested for appropriate patients, as it indicates the patient's ability to discriminate one point from two points when the latter are applied in close proximity. Patients with normal two-point discrimination will also possess good protective sensation and light touch sensation. The problem arises when the patient's response to this test is poor; in that case, the test cannot quantify the patient's level of protective sensation or light touch sensation.

The Semmes-Weinstein monofilaments test is used to quantify the patient's level of light touch sensation and protective sensation. This test should be administered to patients who have had peripheral nerve repair or surgical nerve decompression. The test accurately identifies those areas of the patient's hands that may require special precautions (e.g., thermal gloves) or restrictions from working around moving machinery or in extreme temperatures. The Moberg pick-up test should be used if the patient's job requires manipulation of small objects with vision occluded.

SELECTION OF COORDINATION COMPONENTS

The coordination component is an essential part of the BPCE if the patient must perform activities that require speed and accuracy. The performance of activities of daily living can also be assessed. A patient who labors for a long time in order to perform a coordinated task will frequently avoid use of the injured hand in performing the task. The therapist should select tests that identify the patient's speed, accuracy, and endurance in the performance of work tasks that require coordination.

It is necessary to select the test that will provide the most applicable evaluation. For example, a person with an injury to only one digit, will likely not have difficulty performing activities of daily living. Therefore, a coordination test that focuses on basic prehension skills would not be appropriate. However, for a person with an injury to all digits of the dominant hand, a coordination test of activities of daily living is appropriate. The Jebsen-Taylor Hand Function test is recommended.

If a person's occupation requires speed and accuracy, tests are selected that specifically test those skills. When the physical demands of a person's job require handling, manipulating, and feeling, the Minnesota Rate of Manipulation test, the Purdue Pegboard test, or the Valpar Upper Extremity Range of Motion Work Sample is suggested. When speed of performance is necessary, as in assembly line jobs, the Valpar Simulated Assembly Work Sample is used.

SELECTION OF ENDURANCE TEST COMPONENTS

The objective of evaluating a patient's endurance is to document performance capacity over a prolonged period of time. The patient may perform biomechanical, sensory, and coordination tests within the normal range for a brief period. The same patient, however, may then exhibit muscle fatigue and swelling after repetitive performances of the same test. To evaluate endurance, the therapist selects tasks that simulate physical demands that exist in the patient's daily work requirements and observes the patient performing these tasks for a period of two hours or more. The test should not cause cardiac distress. It is advisable to monitor the patient's vital signs during the endurance evaluation. Indeed, the therapist should not proceed with endurance testing before reviewing the medical documentation for contraindications. Hand volume is measured prior to and after the BPCE. If volume increases more than 50 m.l., it has been the clinical observations that the patient's work perfomance usually is restricted due to pain and edema.

The endurance component of the BPCE is composed of the SPCE, in addition to the BTE work simulator and manual handling tasks. The SPCE is used to evaluate each of the physical demands listed in the *Dictionary of Occupational Titles* (U.S. Dept. of Labor, 1991). Lifting and handling capacity is assessed with the manual handling techniques devised by Snook (1978). Repetitive prolonged manipulation is assessed with standardized manipulation tests that require a prolonged amount of time to administer (Figure 1). Forceful, repetitive tool use is assessed with the BTE Work Simulator (Curtis and Englaitcheff 1981) (Figure 2). Any of these tests should be chosen if an individual's occupational requirements include lifting, carrying, pushing, pulling, handling, and/or manipulating objects for sustained periods.

EQUIPMENT

Equipment necessary for the BPCE includes the following (Resource companies are provided where applicable.):

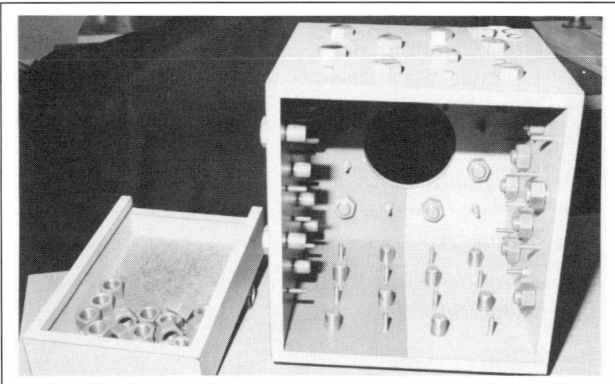

Reprinted with permission from the Hand Rehabilitation Center, Ltd., of Philadelphia, PA

Figure 1　The Valpar Work Samples require prolonged use of the hands for fine manipulation.

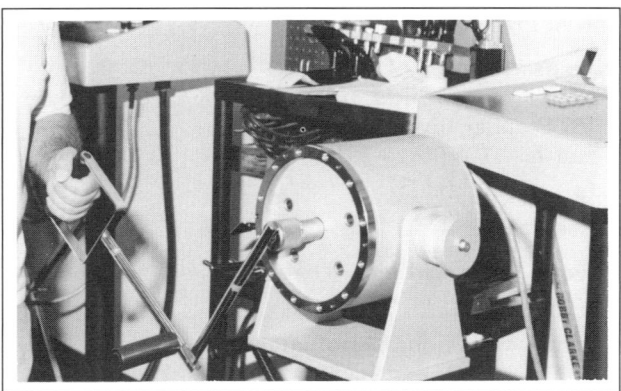

Reprinted with permission from the Hand Rehabilitation Center, Ltd., of Philadelphia, PA

Figure 2　The BTE Work Simulator is used to evaluate the ability to push and pull as is required in the task of sawing.

Bags of gravel (see Chapter 4)

Boley gauge
Volumeters, Unlimited

Box with dowel and slotted handles (see Chapter 4)

Box with side handles
Designed by Susan Smith (see Chapter 2)

Equipment for SPCE (see Chapter 2)

Finger goniometer
BOK
Fred Samons, Incorporated
145 Tower Drive
Burr Ridge, IL 60521

Goniometers for shoulder, elbow, and wrist
J. A. Preston Company
60 Page Road
Clifton, NJ 07012

Hand volumeter
Volumeters Unlimited
52421 Double View Drive
P.O. Box 146
Idlewild, CA 92347

Industrial buckets
Local hardware store
(see Chapter 4)

Jebsen-Taylor Hand Function test
(see Chapter 4)

Milk crates
(see Chapter 4)

Minnesota Rate of Manipulation test
J. A. Preston Corporation

Moberg Pick-Up test
Volumeters, Unlimited

Pinch Gauge
J. A. Preston Corporation

Pipe assembly
North Coast Medical, Inc.
187 Stauffer Blvd.
San Jose, CA 95125-1042

Powers lifting frame
(see Chapter 4)

Purdue Pegboard test
J. A. Preston Corporation

Semmes-Weinstein monofilaments
Volumeters Unlimited

Set of disc weights
Local sporting goods store or
J. A. Preston Corporation

Set of dumbbells (1–25 lb.)
Local sporting goods store or
J. A. Preston Corporation

Stopwatch
Local sporting goods store

Valpar Work Samples
Valpar Corporation
3801 E. 34th Street
Tucson, AZ 85713

Work simulator (lease plan)
Baltimore Therapeutic Equipment Co.
1201 Bernard Drive
Baltimore, MD 21223

Limited space, a problem at many clinics, should not prevent the therapist from offering work-related services. Excellent programs have been carried out in a space as small as 200 square feet. In 1977, the space allotted at the Hand Rehabilitation Center of Philadelphia for administration of physical capacity evaluations and the work tolerance program was 500 square feet. Growth has resulted in 1,200 square feet being used for this service today. At Northeast Work Hardening and Sports Therapy, 5,000 square feet are allocated for hand therapy and work hardening use.

No matter what size floor space, the therapist should be careful to arrange the equipment so as to prevent accidents. The individual being tested must be able to lift and carry objects without harming other patients.

ADMINISTRATION OF TESTS

Administration of each test component should be done exactly as specified by the authors in the administration manual or reference. For illustration of the patient's participation, a brief summary of the test administration is provided.

Biomechanical Tests

To test muscle strength of isolated muscles or groups of muscles, the therapist should use the techniques described by Kendall and McCreary (1983).

To measure joint range of motion, use the standard methods of measuring with a goniometer as described by the American Academy of Orthopedic Surgeons (1965).

To measure isometric pinch strength, Mathiowetz et al. (1985) required subjects to sit with their shoulder adducted and neutrally rotated, elbow flexed at 90 degrees, forearm in neutral and wrist between 0 degrees and 15 degrees ulnar deviation. The B&L pinch gauge (B&L Engineering Co., 12309 East Florence, Santa Fe Springs, CA 90670) is used to measure tip pinch, three-point pinch and key pinch. Three successive trials are recorded. The right hand is tested first, then the left hand, for each pinch pattern. The mean of the trials is the test score.

To measure isometric grip strength, the standardized method of positioning the patient as described by Mathiowetz et al. (1985) is used. The therapist should hold the Jamar dynamometer (J.A. Preston, Co., 60 Page Road, Clifton, NJ 07012) around the readout dial. The patient is asked to squeeze the handle, which is set on the second handle position, three successive times. The mean score is recorded.

To measure exertion of maximal effort on the isometric grip test, the patient is tested on the Jamar dynamometer set at each of the five handle positions as described by Stokes (1983). The patient's one-time maximum exertion for each level is charted on the graph. The uninjured hand is tested prior to testing the injured hand.

To evaluate isometric grip strength with the BTE

Work Simulator, standard methods developed by Berlin and Vermette (1985) are used. The Work Simulator shaft is positioned at the elbow crease of the standing subject, and the grip attachment (#162) is inserted into the shaft. The subject's hand is placed on the grip attachment and the placement of the web space is marked. The dominant hand is tested first. The subject is instructed to squeeze the grip attachment twice through the full range of motion at 20 in./lb. of resistance to warm up. Then the subject applies maximum isometric force three times, relaxing the grip between each effort. The test is repeated with the nondominant hand. The mean of the three scores for each hand is recorded.

To evaluate power or dynamic grip strength, Berlin and Vermette suggested the patient stand in the same position as for the isometric grip strength test. The resistance is set at one-half of the lowest isometric torque (in./lb.) score for both hands. The subject squeezes the grip attachment in and out as rapidly as possible for 10 seconds. The mean of three scores is recorded.

Sensibility Tests

To evaluate static two-point discrimination, the patient is seated, with the hand positioned palm up on a form-fitting mold of putty, and with vision occluded. The therapist lightly applies either one or two points to a fingertip, without blanching the skin. Points should be applied longitudinally, parallel to the phalanx. The patient is asked whether he or she felt one or two points. The procedure is repeated on each fingertip, starting within the normal range of 5 mm. If the patient cannot accurately identify the number of points in 7 out of 10 trials, the points are moved further apart 1 mm at a time, up to 15 mm maximum (Callahan 1984).

To evaluate moving two-point discrimination, the patient is seated and positioned as with the static two-point discrimination task. The therapist applies one or two points transversely to the fingertip, moving the instrument from proximal to distal. The test starts with two points at 2 mm. apart, increasing the distance 1 mm. at a time. The separation should increase to 5 mm. if the patient can accurately identify the number of points in 7 out of 10 trials (Dellon 1981).

Light touch/deep pressure is evaluated with Semmes-Weinstein monofilaments according to the method described by Callahan (1984). The patient is positioned in the same way as during the two-point discrimination task (Figure 3). Starting with size 2.83 filament and progressing to heavier filaments, the therapist continues applying the filaments, three

times each, up to the size 4.17 filament. All filaments above this size are applied only once. The filaments are applied with the lightest pressure necessary to bend or bow the filament slightly (Figure 4). The time of application is 1.5 seconds. Testing proceeds until the patient can identify correctly when he or she is touched two out of three times. Both hands are tested on the volar and dorsal surfaces.

To evaluate localization ability, tactile gnosis, and speed of prehension with vision occluded, the Moberg Pick-Up test is administered. The patient is timed while using each hand separately to pick up any seven objects (e.g., coin, pin, safety pin, nut, bolt, piece of fabric, cotton ball) and place them in a box with each hand separately. A screen is placed on the table, and the patient, with vision blocked, is timed while picking up the seven objects again with each hand (Sunderland 1978).

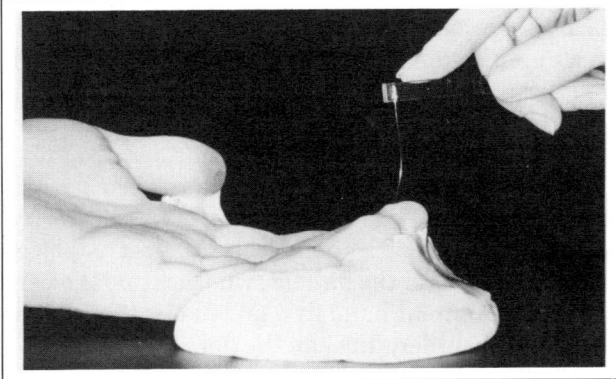

Reprinted with permission from the Hand Rehabilitation Center, Ltd., of Philadelphia, PA

Figure 3 The patient's hand is positioned on a mound of putty to prevent vibration.

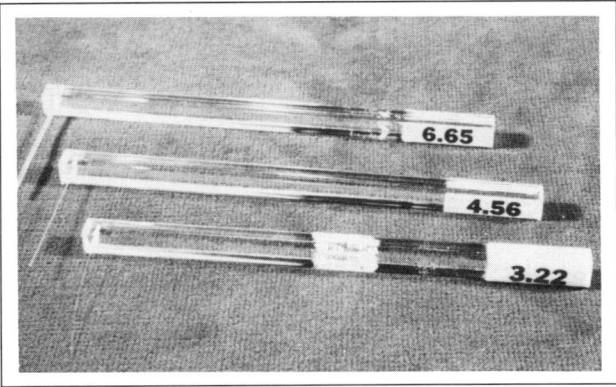

Reprinted with permission from the Hand Rehabilitation Center, Ltd., of Philadelphia, PA

Figure 4 The Semmes-Weinstein Monofilaments are applied for 1.5 seconds until each one bows.

Coordination Tests

The Purdue Pegboard test is used to evaluate fingertip dexterity. The patient sits at a table 30-inches high. The pegboard is directly in front of the patient (Figure 5). For the first test, the patient uses the dominant hand to place as many pins as possible, one at a time, into the row on the pegboard closest to the hand. The patient is stopped after 30 seconds. The non-dominant hand is then evaluated with the same procedure. The total number of pins placed in the row is used as the patient's score. Exact instructions should be read to the patient from the *Purdue Pegboard Administration Manual* during the test adminstration (Tiffin 1968).

Next, the patient uses both hands to pick up the pins and place them in the two rows on the pegboard. The patient is stopped after 30 seconds, and the pins are counted. For the assembly test, the patient picks up a pin from the right hand cup and places it in the top hole in the right-hand row. As the left hand picks up a washer and places it on the pin, the right hand picks up a collar and places it over the washer. Finally, the left hand picks up a washer and places it over the collar. The patient is stopped after one minute and the number of pieces assembled are counted.

The Nine Hole Peg test was developed by Mathiowetz et al.(1984) for evaluation of fine dexterity. The patient sits at a table. The Peg test is placed directly in front of the patient, who picks up the pegs with the dominant hand first and places them in the holes, in any order, until all the holes are filled (Figure 6). The patient then removes the pegs (one at a time) until all pegs are removed. The timing is stopped when the patient removes the last peg and places it in the storage container.

The Jebsen-Taylor Hand Function test is administered to patients who report diminished capacity to perform activities of daily living (Jebsen et al. 1969). There are seven subtests. The specific instructions for each sub-test should be read to the patient, who is seated at a table and performs each subtest as follows:

1. Writes a sentence on an 8½″ × 11″ white paper with a ball point pen, while reading the typed sentence from an 8″ × 5″ index card. The patient is timed while writing with each hand (Figure 7).
2. Turns 5″ × 7″ cards over by reaching across his or her mid-line with each hand separately. The time is recorded.
3. Is timed while picking up, with each hand, two paper clips, two bottle caps, and two pennies, one at a time, and placing them in an empty one-pound coffee can.

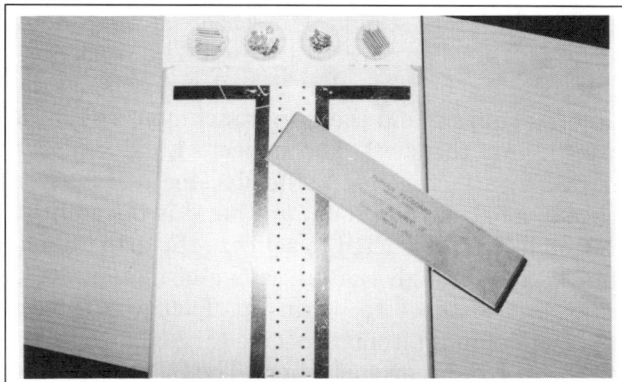

Reprinted with permission from the Hand Rehabilitation Center, Ltd., of Philadelphia, PA

Figure 5   The Purdue Pegboard is administered to patients whose jobs require fine fingertip dexterity.

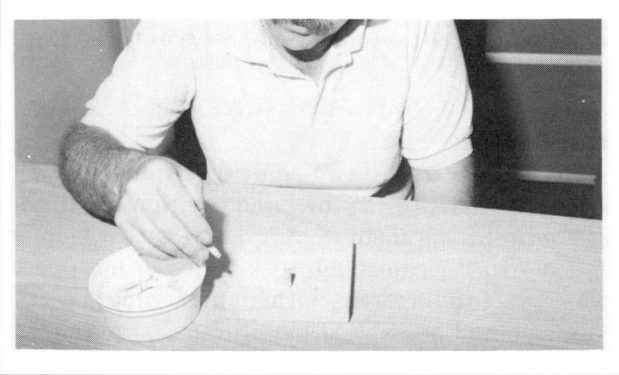

Reprinted with permission from the Hand Rehabilitation Center, Ltd., of Philadelphia, PA

Figure 6   The patient is required to place and remove pegs from the test as rapidly as possible.

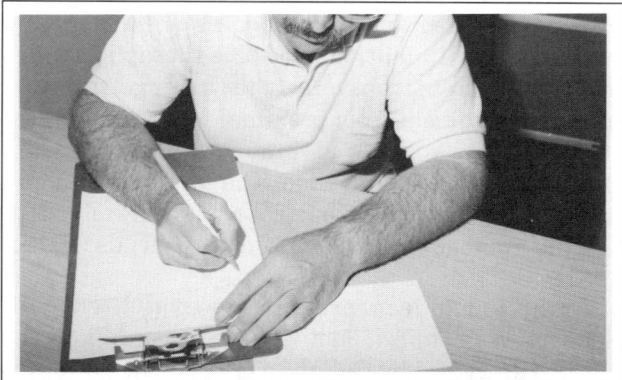

Reprinted with permission from the Hand Rehabilitation Center, Ltd., of Philadelphia, PA

Figure 7   Writing is evaluated with the Jebsen-Taylor Hand Function Test

4. Picks up five beans with a teaspoon, one at a time from the test board, and places them in a one-pound coffee can.
5. Is timed while stacking four checkers onto the test board.
6. Lifts five empty one-pound cans onto the test board (Figure 8).
7. Is timed while lifting full one-pound cans onto the test board (Figures 9, 10).

The Minnesota Rate of Manipulation test is selected for evaluation of reaching and handling ability. For instructions for the 32023(4207) Minnesota Manual Dexterity test, write Lafayette Instrument Company, P.O. Box 5729, Lafayette, IN 47903. There are two tests utilized in the BPCE. In both tests the patient is seated with the test board directly in front on the table. In the Placing test, the patient moves the blocks from the far side of the board to the near side. The instructions from the administration manual should be read verbatim to the patient. The patient is timed while completing the Placing test four times with each hand. The scores are added for a total score (Figure 11). In the Turning test, the patient picks up a block with the left hand and then turns it over and places it in the hole on the board with the right hand. The total time of the four trials is calculated (Figure 12).

The Valpar Work Samples are designed to test specific physical demands as defined in the *Dictionary of Occupational Titles* (U.S. Dept. of Labor 1991). Selection of which test to use depends upon the patient's job demands. The Valpar Work Samples are chosen to evaluate reaching, handling, and manipulating while working in various body postures (Baxter and McEntee 1984). Administration of each work sample should be in accordance with the instructions in the administration manual (Valpar).

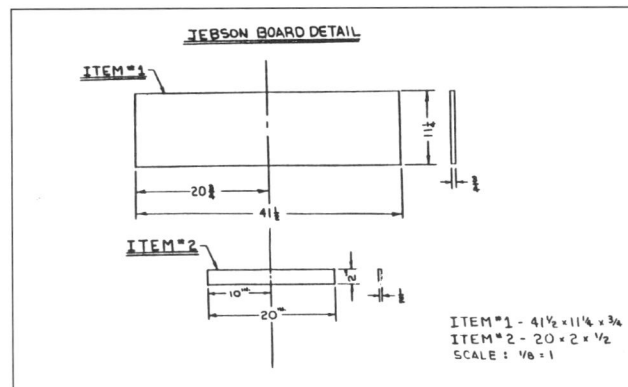

Reprinted with permission from the Hand Rehabilitation Center, Ltd., of Philadelphia, PA

Figure 9 The board for the Jebsen-Taylor Hand Function Test has two surfaces.

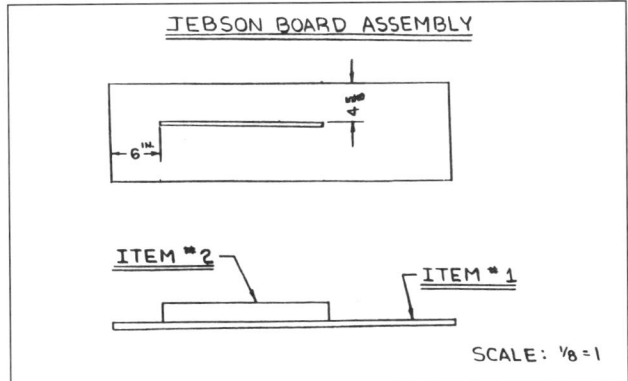

Reprinted with permission from the Hand Rehabilitation Center, Ltd., of Philadelphia, PA

Figure 10 The perpendicular surface prevents the objects from moving beyond the patient's reach.

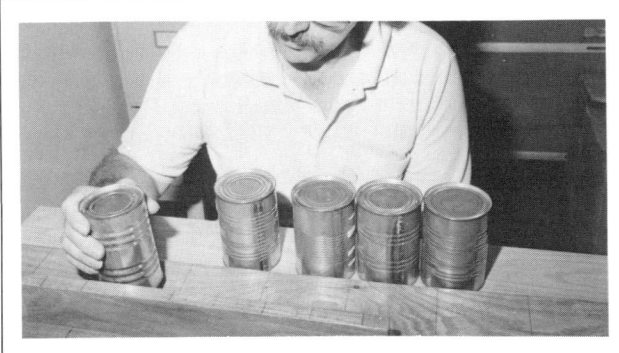

Reprinted with permission from the Hand Rehabilitation Center, Ltd., of Philadelphia, PA

Figure 8 Cans are lifted from the table and placed on the test board.

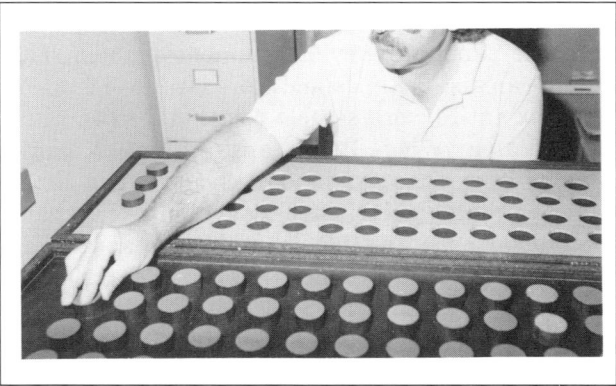

Reprinted with permission from the Hand Rehabilitation Center, Ltd., of Philadelphia, PA

Figure 11 In the placing test, the patient reaches out to move the objects closer to him.

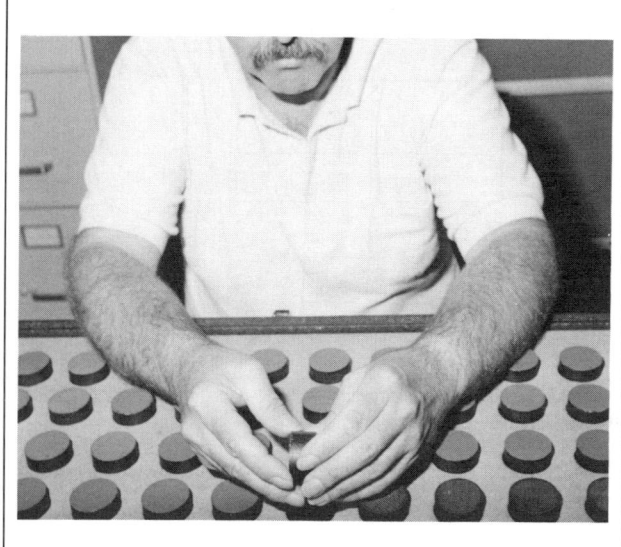

Figure 12 Bilateral gross hand and arm movements are required for completion of the turning test.

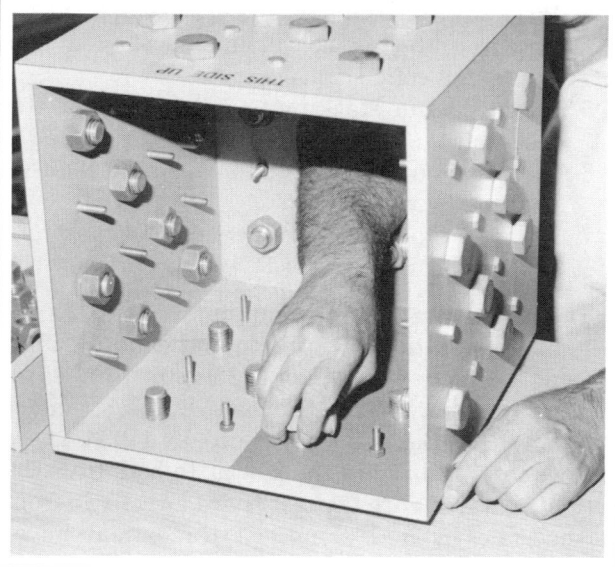

Figure 13 The patient reaches through the circular holes to place nuts on the bolts inside the Valpar Upper Extremity Range of Motion Work Sample.

For the Valpar Upper Extremity Range of Motion Work Sample, the two components of the work sample are placed directly in front of the patient who is seated at a table. The patient uses the right hand to place the nuts on the four panels on the left side of the work sample. The patient is timed until each panel is completed. Then, the left hand is timed for each panel completed on the right side of the box. The scores are added for each hand (Figure 13).

The Valpar Small Tools Mechanical Work Sample is useful for evaluating the patient's tool handling ability. In each of the five sections, the patient is scored separately while using tools to assemble small nuts and bolts on each panel. The therapist may score one panel only, or any number of them. The patient can also be timed and scored while disassembling the entire work sample box (Figure 14).

The Valpar Whole Body Range of Motion Work Sample requires the patient to reach and handle three plexiglass plates while fastening and removing them from four panels. The panels are located at various heights which require reaching overhead, bending, and stooping (Figures 15, 16).

The Valpar Simulated Assembly Work Sample simulates assembly tasks in several industrial jobs. The patient stands and picks up a pin with the right hand and a black and a white plastic part with the left hand. The patient places the pin in the rotating wheel, then places the black part and then the white

part onto the pin. The task can be accomplished by using either hand. The assembly continues for 20 minutes, and the score is based on the total number of correct assemblies (Figure 17).

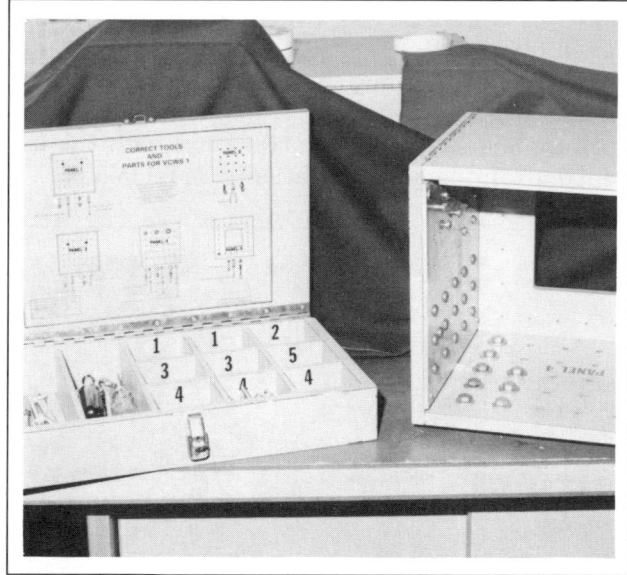

Figure 14 Common tools, such as wrenches, pliers and screwdrivers are used to assemble the Valpar Small Tools Work Sample.

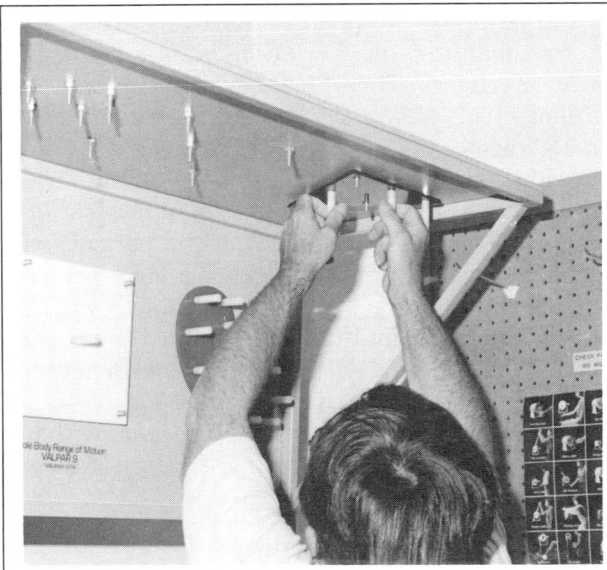

Reprinted with permission from the Hand Rehabilitation Center, Ltd., of Philadelphia, PA

Figure 15 Reaching overhead is required, as well as manipulation of nuts onto bolts to secure the plexiglass plates onto each panel.

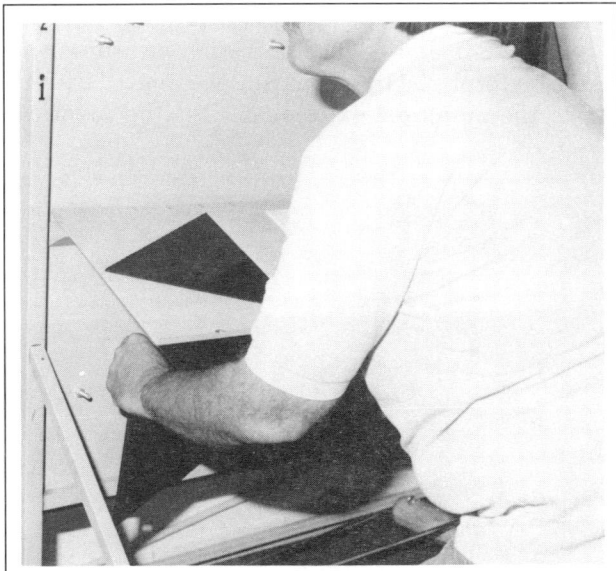

Reprinted with permission from the Hand Rehabilitation Center, Ltd., of Philadelphia, PA

Figure 16 Bending and stooping is evaluated as well as reaching, handling and manipulating.

Endurance Tests

The SPCE is used to evaluate the patient's ability to perform the 20 physical demands as described in Chapter 2. The Minnesota Rate of Manipulation test, the Valpar Upper Extremity Range of Motion Work Sample, the Valpar Simulated Assembly Work Sample, the Valpar Small Tools Mechanical Work Sample, and the Valpar Whole Body Range of Motion Work Sample are used to evaluate the patient's endurance in the performance of tasks that involve reaching, handling and manipulating.

Snook's (1978) method is recommended for evaluating the patient's manual handling and lifting capacities. Snook instructed subjects to lift a weighted box from floor height to knuckle height, then from knuckle height to shoulder height, and finally from shoulder height to arm's reach overhead. The weight in the box was controlled by the subjects. Snook noted that subjects tended to lift the initial weight that was given to them. Therefore, to determine each subject's maximum acceptable weight, two trials were performed. In the first trial, the subject was given a box with a very heavy weight and was instructed to make adjustments in the weight. During the second trial, the subject was given a box with a very light weight and was encouraged to add weight to the maximum acceptable level. If the results of the two trials were within 15% of each other in weight, the average of the two results were recorded. In Snook's research, the subjects also performed repetitive lifting of the maximum acceptable weight for longer periods of time after they had participated in a five-day conditioning program.

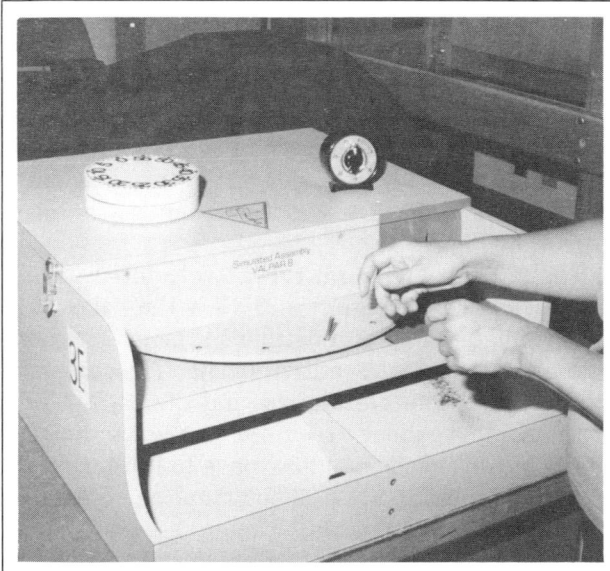

Reprinted with permission from the Hand Rehabilitation Center, Ltd., of Philadelphia, PA

Figure 17 Repetitive assembly requiring rapid hand use can be assessed on the Valpar Simulated Assembly Work Sample.

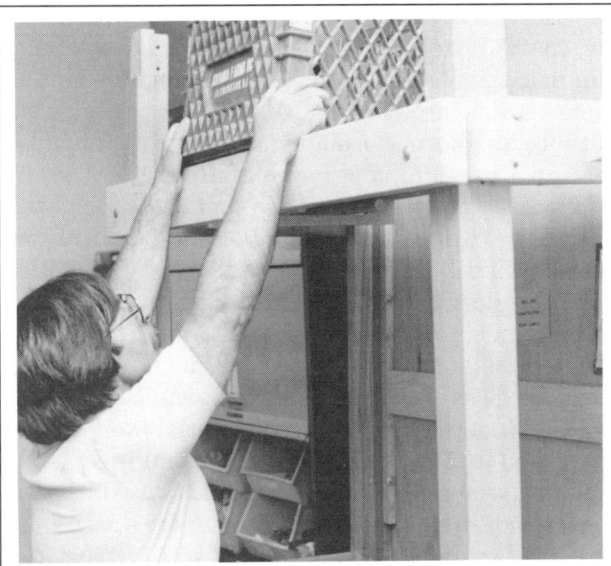

Reprinted with permission from the Hand Rehabilitation Center, Ltd., of Philadelphia, PA

Figure 18 The Powers Lifting Frame is adjustable to enable the patient to reach arm's length to an overhead shelf.

The lifting evaluation of the BPCE utilizes Snook's method for lifting to various heights. The patient places a 10-lb. weight in the SPCE box with side handles, or in a milk crate, and lifts the box or crate from the floor to the shelf of the Powers lifting frame at knuckle height. Then, the patient returns the box to the floor and adds weight. The process is continued until the patient cannot lift heavier weight without risk of injury. After the patient is allowed to rest for two minutes, the lifting test is conducted from knuckle height to shoulder height. A very heavy amount of weight is placed in the box, and the patient unloads it to his or her maximum acceptable weight. The final lifting test is performed in the same manner from shoulder height to the patient's arm reach overhead (Figure 18).

The amount of weight repetitively lifted during the test is usually significantly less than the maximum weight lifted at any time on the job for those whose job requires repetitive lifting. The submaximal weight is placed in a box and the patient lifts at the same frequency required on the job. For example, a warehouseman may have to lift one 50-lb. box per minute at work. (The actual amount to be lifted is determined from a job analysis—see Chapter 5). During the BPCE, this patient would lift a 50-lb. box once a minute continually and would be timed to determine endurance. The patient is instructed to stop before becoming strained or fatigued.

To evaluate endurance related to repetitive, forceful tool handling, the Work Simulator is the instrument of choice. Those tools which simulate the patient's tools at work are used. If a patient drives an 18-wheeler diesel truck, the steering wheel tool attachment is inserted in the shaft of the brake mechanism (Figure 19). The resistance is set at a comfortable level determined by the patient, who turns the steering wheel with each hand separately until beginning to feel tired. To calculate power output, the computer multiplies the applied force by the distance the steering wheel is turned and divides the result by the time the patient works. The powers of each hand are compared. Testing continues with numerous tools to evaluate the power output for each work activity (Figure 20).

RATING AND INTERPRETATION

Interpretation of the patient's test performance is based on comparison of the patient's ratings on all the tests administered. Ratings vary among tests. For example, the patient's performance on the SPCE is rated on a developmental scale for age and sex. The manual muscle test is rated by grade according to the strength of each muscle (Kendall and McCreary 1983). Joint range of motion measurements can be interpreted by comparing the injured extremity to the uninjured extremity. Also, the American

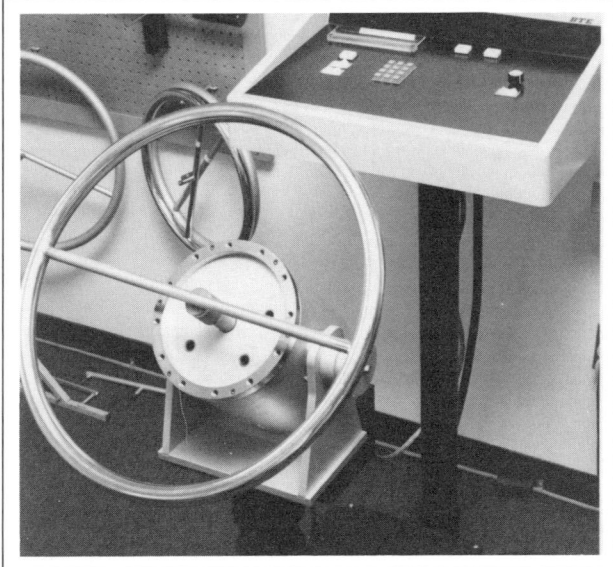

Reprinted with permission from the Hand Rehabilitation Center, Ltd., of Philadelphia, PA

Figure 19 The patient sits in front of the brake mechanism and steers the tool attachment (# 141) against resistance set at a submaximal level.

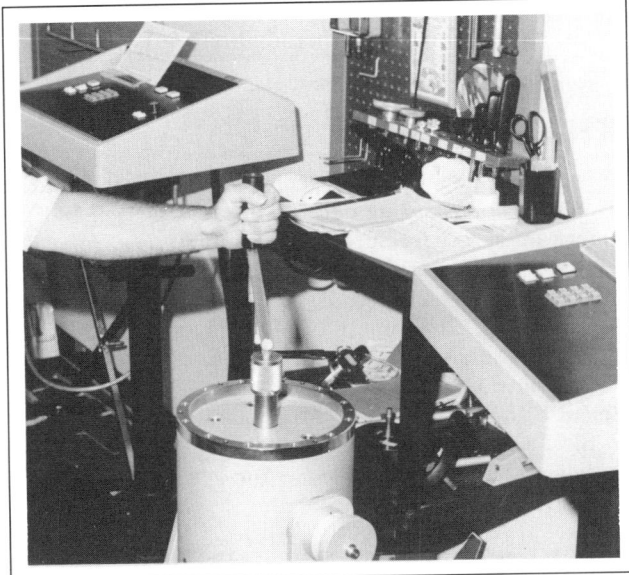

Reprinted with permission from the Hand Rehabilitation Center, Ltd., of Philadelphia, PA

Figure 20 A truck driver may use this motion to shift gears. Both hands are tested and the power output of each hand is compared.

Academy of Orthopedic Surgeons (1965) has defined ranges within which specific joints move. The Clinical Assessment Committee of the American Society for Surgery of the Hand (1978) defines the acceptable quality of two point discrimination by the hand. The quality of light touch/deep pressure was arbitrarily assigned to the Semmes-Weinstein monofilaments by Bell. (1984). Stokes (1983) evaluated the patient's maximum exertion by graphing the result of a grip test recorded for each handle position. He found that all patients, even the unconditioned ones, would demonstrate a bell-shaped curve in their measurements when exerting their maximum effort.

In research on manual handling tasks, Snook (1978) found that there was no single maximum weight that could be lifted by all patients. Therefore, the average of two trials is recorded if the weights are within 15 percent of each other for each trial. If the weights are not within 15 percent of each other, the patient is asked to lift more weight during additional trials.

Berlin and Vermette (1985) developed norms for static (force) and dynamic (power) grip strength measured on the Work Simulator for dominant and nondominant hands. Tables 1 and 2* illustrate the male

* Tables are included at the end of this chapter.

and female mean force and power output, as well as the percentiles into which the scores fall.

Standardized test results are interpreted by percentiles that can be used to compare the injured worker to the uninjured population. The Valpar Upper Extremity Range of Motion Work Sample, the Valpar Whole Body Range of Motion Work Sample, the Purdue Pegboard, and the Minnesota Rate of Manipulation test scores are grouped into the following percentiles: 75% and above indicates above average ability and excellent potential for the worker to compete with the uninjured population; 60–75% indicates adequate ability to compete in the workplace; and less than 60% indicates below average ability of the injured worker to compete with the uninjured population.

Interpretation of standardized tests that are scored on the basis of method-timed motion standards require a different interpretation. Method-timed motion standards were developed by industrial engineers to set quotas for minimum production rates. Scores range from 0 to 150%. The Valpar Corporation has suggested that patients who score 100% or better can qualify for entry-level work and are likely to perform at a level that will promote and maintain their jobs. The Valpar Simulated Assembly Work Sample and the Valpar Small Tools Mechanical Work Samples are scored in accordance with method-timed motion standards.

Standardized test scores may also be interpreted on the basis of standard deviations. Standard deviations are used to interpret the static and dynamic grip strength test on the Work Simulator (Tables 1, 2), the Jebsen-Taylor Hand Function test (Tables 3–6*); and the grip test, pinch test, and Nine-Hole Peg test by Mathiowetz (Tables 7–12*). The therapist reports that the patient is functioning within normal limits if the score is not less than two standard deviations lower than the mean score.

Depending on the length of the BPCE, the therapist may select the standardized test to augment the amount of information relevant to determining the patient's ability to perform a specific job. The therapist must select standardized tests carefully, however, as their administration requires various lengths of time and adds significantly to the total time of the evaluation. The number of standardized tests during the four-hour evaluation is usually limited to two or three. When all the test scores are computed, the therapist should check for the patient's maximum physical ability. Coefficient of variance is calculated on the static grip test of the BTE Work Simulator to check for consistent effort by the patient (Berlin and Vermette, 1985). The therapist should state whether the patient appeared to exert maximum effort on all tests.

The patient's maximum physical abilities are compared to the job requirements. If the patient can perform a large majority of the physical demands of the job, but is unable to perform one or two tasks, the employer should be contacted. If the employer can arrange assistance for those few tasks the injured worker cannot perform, the patient can return to the regular job.

If there are several tasks the patient cannot perform, the employer should be contacted. Arrangement of a modified job requirements is feasible in many industrial settings. Also, an arrangement for part-time work or job rotation may be helpful. In a job rotation arrangement, the injured worker may work part of the day on the regular job and part of the day on a job that is less physically stressful.

There are times when the patient cannot return to a former place of employment. The BPCE outlines all the patient's physical abilities and restrictions. The report is sent to the patient's vocational counselor, vocational placement specialist, or new employer. In cases of litigation, the BPCE should include detailed descriptions of the patient's physical capacities and limitations related to performance of all occupational activities including work, play, and self-maintenance.

REPORTING

The findings of the BPCE are composed into a narrative report or an abbreviated short form with a summary. The majority of the time, the narrative report is produced, as the contents are complete and easily understood by any one of the referral sources. Completed narrative reports and abbreviated reports are included in Chapter 8.

The therapist summarizes the patient's test response in the final section of the report, entitled "Summary and Recommendations." In addition to the test response, the therapist should include recommendations concerning the feasibility for the patient's occupational placement. It is imperative that a definite recommendation be made stating the patient's ability to work at his or her former job, a modified job, or a classification of specific level of work as described in the *Dictionary of Occupational Titles* (U.S. Dept. of Labor, 1977). Any recommendations for adaptive equipment or protective clothing should be stated. Also, if the patient's schedule

for working is to be modified, recommendations for modification should be included as well.

REFERENCES

American Academy of Orthopedic Surgeons. *Joint Motion, Method of Measuring and Recording*, Chicago: 1965.

American Society for Surgery of the Hand. *The Hand Examination and Diagnosis*, Colorado: 1978

Baxter, P. and McEntee, P. M. "The Physical Capacity Evaluation," In Hunter, J. M., Schneider, L., Mackin, E. and Callahan, A. (Eds.) *Rehabilitation of the Hand.* St. Louis: C.V. Mosby, 1984.

Berlin, S., and Vermette, J. "An Exploratory Study of Work Simulator Norms for Grip and Wrist Flexion," *Vocational Evaluation and Work Adjustment Bulletin* (Summer, 1985):61–5.

Callahan, A. D. "Sensibility Testing: Clinical Methods." In Hunter, J.M., Schneider, L., Mackin, E., and Callahan, A. (Eds.) *Rehabilitation of the Hand.* St. Louis: C.V. Mosby, 1984, pp. 407-31.

Curtis, R. M. and Englaitcheff, J. "A Work Simulator for Rehabilitating the Upper Extremity—Preliminary Report," *Journal of Hand Surgery* 6 (1981): 499–501.

Dellon, A. L. *Evaluation of Sensibility and Re-education of Sensation in the Hand.* Baltimore: Williams and Wilkins, 1981.

Gill, T. and Trujillo, S. A. "The Minnesota Rate of Manipulation Test: A Reliability Test Among Psychiatric Clients in a Sheltered Workshop." *Vocational Evaluation and Work Adjustment Bulletin* (Fall 1985): 108–13.

Jebsen, R. H., Taylor, N., Trieschmann, R. B., Trotter, M.J., and Howard, L.A. "An Objective and Standardized Test of Hand Function." *Archives of Physical Medicine and Rehabilitation* 50 (1969): 311–19.

Kendall, F. P. and McCreary, E. K. *Muscle Testing and Function*, Third Edition, Baltimore: Williams and Wilkins, 1983.

Mathiowetz, V., Kashman, N. Volland, G., Weber, K., Dowe, M., and Rogers, S. "Grip and Pinch Strength: Normative Data for Adults," *Archives of Physical Medicine and Rehabilitation* 66 (February 1985) 69–74.

Mathiowetz, V., Weber, K., Bolland, G., and Kashman, N. "Reliability and Validity of Hand Strength Evaluation." *Journal of Hand Surgery* 9a (1984): 222–26.

Snook, S. H. "The Design of Manual Handling Tasks" *Ergonomics*, 21 (1978) 963–85.

Stokes, H. M. "The Seriously Uninjured Hand—Weakness of Grip," *Journal of Occupational Medicine* 25 (September, 1983).

Sunderland, S. *Nerves and Nerve Injuries.* (2d ed). New York: Churchill Livingstone, 1978.

Tiffin, J. *Purdue Pegboard Examiner Manual.* Chicago. Science Research Associates, 1968.

U.S. Dept. of Labor. *Dictionary of Occupational Titles*, Fourth Edition: Washington, DC: U.S. Government Printing Office, 1991.

MALE STATIC GRIP STRENGTH
Tool #161

Dominant

inch/lbs.	percentile
551	99
530	98
500	96
470	93
440	89
std. dev. 419	84
380	74
350	63
mean 320	50
290	37
260	26
std. dev. 221	16
200	11
170	7
140	4
110	2
89	1
std. dev.	99

Non-Dominant

inch/lbs.	percentile
502	99
479	98
449	96
419	91
std. dev. 386	84
359	75
329	63
mean 299	50
269	37
239	25
std. dev. 212	16
179	9
149	4
119	2
96	1
std. dev.	87

FEMALE STATIC GRIP STRENGTH
Tool #161

Dominant

inch/lbs.	percentile
285	99
265	97
245	92
std. dev. 228	84
225	82
205	68
mean 185	50
165	32
145	18
std. dev. 142	16
125	8
105	3
85	1
std. dev.	43

Non-Dominant

inch/lbs.	percentile
238	99
232	98
222	96
212	92
202	86
std. dev. 200	84
192	76
182	64
mean 172	50
162	36
152	24
std. dev. 144	16
142	14
132	8
122	4
112	2
106	1
std. dev.	28

MALE DYNAMIC GRIP POWER
Tool #161

Dominant

engals	percentile
17098	99
15721	97
14721	93
13721	86
std. dev. 13458	84
12721	77
11721	64
mean 10721	50
9721	36
8721	23
std. dev. 7984	16
7721	14
6721	7
5721	3
4344	1
std. dev.	2737

Non-Dominant

engals	percentile
16095	99
15032	97
14032	94
13032	87
std. dev. 12634	84
12032	78
11032	65
mean 10032	50
9032	35
8032	22
std. dev. 7430	16
7032	13
6032	6
5032	3
3959	1
std. dev.	2602

FEMALE DYNAMIC GRIP POWER
Tool #161

Dominant

engals	percentile
8999	99
8725	98
8225	96
7725	92
7225	86
std. dev. 7130	84
6725	76
6225	68
mean 5725	50
5225	32
4725	24
std. dev. 4320	16
4225	14
3725	8
3225	4
2725	2
2451	1
std. dev.	1405

Non-Dominant

engals	percentile
9011	99
8507	98
8007	95
7507	91
std. dev. 7011	84
6507	75
6007	63
mean 5507	50
5007	37
4507	25
std. dev. 4003	16
3507	9
3007	5
2507	2
2003	1
std. dev.	1504

Tables 1.2

Male and female grip strength measurements can be interpreted by either the mean and standard deviation, or the percentiles available through the research of Berlin and Vermette.

Reprinted with permission from the *Vocational Evaluation and Work Adjustment Bulletin*, July 1985

45

TABLE 3

JEBSEN-TAYLOR HAND FUNCTION TEST (Males, ages 20--59)

DOMINATE HAND

TASK	NORM	X+ 2 S.D.
WRITING	12.2 ± 3.5	19.2
CARDS	4.0 ± 0.9	5.8
SMALL OBJECTS	5.0 ± 1.0	7.0
EATING	$6.4 \pm$	8.2
CHECKERS	$3.3 \pm$	4.7
EMPTY CANS	$3.0 \pm$	3.8
FULL CANS	$3.0 \pm$	4.0

NON-DOMINATE HAND

TASK	NORM	X+ 2 S.D.
WRITING	32.3 ± 11.8	55.0
CARDS	$4.5 \pm$	6.3
SMALL OBJECTS	$6.2 \pm$	8.0
EATING	$7.0 \pm$	10.5
CHECKERS	$3.8 \pm$	5.0
EMPTY CANS	$3.2 \pm$	4.4
FULL CANS	$3.1 \pm$	3.9

(Reprinted with Permission from the Archives of Physical Medicine and Rehabilitation, Volume 50, June 1969.)

TABLE 4

JEBSEN-TAYLOR HAND FUNCTION TEST (Males, ages 60--94)

DOMINATE HAND

TASK	NORM	X+ 2 S.D.
WRITING	19.5 ± 7.5	34.5
CARDS	5.3 ± 1.6	8.5
SMALL OBJECTS	6.8 ± 1.2	9.2
EATING	6.9 ± 0.9	8.7
CHECKERS	3.8 ± 0.7	5.2
EMPTY CANS	3.6 ± 0.7	5.8
FULL CANS	3.5 ± 0.7	4.9

NON-DOMINATE HAND

TASK	NORM	X+ 2 S.D.
WRITING	48.2 ± 19.1	86.4
CARDS	6.1 ± 2.2	10.5
SMALL OBJECTS	7.9 ± 1.9	11.7
EATING	8.6 ± 1.5	11.6
CHECKERS	4.6 ± 1.0	6.6
EMPTY CANS	3.9 ± 5.3	5.3
FULL CANS	3.8 ± 0.7	5.2

(Reprinted with Permission from the Archives of Physical Medicine and Rehabilitation, Volume 50, June 1969.)

TABLE 5

JEBSEN-TAYLOR HAND FUNCTION TEST (Females, ages 20--59)

DOMINATE HAND

TASK	NORM	X+ 2 S.D.
WRITING	11.7 ± 2.1	15.9
CARDS	4.3 ± 1.4	7.1
SMALL OBJECTS	5.5 ± 0.8	7.1
EATING	6.7 ± 1.1	8.9
CHECKERS	3.3 ± 0.6	4.5
EMPTY CANS	3.1 ± 0.5	4.1
FULL CANS	3.2 ± 0.5	4.2

NON-DOMINATE HAND

TASK	NORM	X+ 2 S.D.
WRITING	30.2 ± 8.6	47.4
CARDS	4.8 ± 1.1	7.0
SMALL OBJECTS	6.0 ± 1.0	8.0
EATING	8.0 ± 1.6	11.2
CHECKERS	3.8 ± 0.7	5.2
EMPTY CANS	3.3 ± 0.6	4.5
FULL CANS	3.3 ± 0.5	4.3

(Reprinted with Permission from the Archives of Physical Medicine and Rehabilitation, Volume 50, June 1969.)

TABLE 6

JEBSEN-TAYLOR HAND FUNCTION TEST (Females, ages 60-94)

DOMINATE HAND

TASK	NORM	X+ 2 S.D.
WRITING	15.7 ± 4.7	25.1
CARDS	4.9 ± 1.2	7.3
SMALL OBJECTS	6.6 ± 1.3	9.2
EATING	6.8 ± 1.1	9.0
CHECKERS	3.6 ± 0.6	4.8
EMPTY CANS	3.5 ± 0.6	4.7
FULL CANS	3.5 ± 0.6	4.7

NON-DOMINATE HAND

TASK	NORM	X+ 2 S.D.
WRITING	38.9 ± 14.9	68.7
CARDS	$.5.5 \pm 1.1$	7.7
SMALL OBJECTS	6.6 ± 0.8	8.2
EATING	8.7 ± 2.0	12.7
CHECKERS	4.4 ± 1.0	6.4
EMPTY CANS	3.4 ± 0.6	4.6
FULL CANS	3.7 ± 0.7	5.1

(Reprinted with Permission from the Archives of Physical Medicine and Rehabilitation, Volume 50, June 1969.)

TABLE 7

AVERAGE PERFORMANCE OF NORMAL MALES ON GRIP STRENGTH (Pounds)

Age	Hand	Mean*	SD	SE	LOW	HIGH
20-24	R	121.0	20.6	3.8	91	167
	L	104.5	21.8	4.0	71	150
25-29	R	120.8	23.0	4.4	78	158
	L	110.5	16.2	3.1	77	139
30-34	R	121.8	22.4	4.3	70	170
	L	110.4	21.7	4.2	64	145
35-39	R	119.7	24.0	4.8	76	176
	L	112.9	21.7	4.4	73	157
40-44	R	116.8	20.7	4.1	84	165
	L	112.8	18.7	3.7	73	157
45-49	R	109.9	23.0	4.3	65	155
	L	100.8	22.8	4.3	58	160
50-54	R	113.6	18.1	3.6	79	151
	L	101.9	17.0	3.4	70	143
55-59	R	101.1	26.7	5.8	59	154
	L	83.2	23.4	5.1	43	128
60-64	R	89.7	20.4	4.2	51	137
	L	76.8	20.3	4.1	27	116
65-69	R	19.1	20.6	4.0	56	131
	L	76.8	19.8	3.8	43	117
70-74	R	75.3	21.5	4.2	32	108
	L	64.8	18.1	3.7	32	93
75+	R	65.7	21.0	4.2	40	135
	L	55.0	17.0	3.4	31	119
All Male	R	104.3	28.3	1.6	32	176
Subjects	L	93.1	27.6	1.6	27	160

* The above mean scores for older subjects may be slightly low (0-10 pounds lower than they should be) due to instrument error detected after the study

Reprinted with permission from the Archives of Physical Medicine and Rehabilitation, Volume 66. February 1985

TABLE 8

AVERAGE PERFORMANCE OF NORMAL FEMALES ON GRIP STRENGTH (Pounds)

Age	Hand	Mean*	SD	SE	Low	High
20-24	R	70.4	14.5	2.8	46	95
	L	61.0	13.1	2.6	33	88
25-29	R	74.5	13.9	2.7	48	97
	L	63.5	12.2	2.4	48	97
30-34	R	78.7	19.2	3.8	46	137
	L	68.0	17.7	3.5	36	115
35-39	R	74.1	10.8	2.2	50	99
	L	66.3	11.7	2.3	49	91
40-44	R	70.4	13.5	2.4	38	103
	L	62.3	13.8	2.5	35	94
45-49	R	62.2	15.1	3.0	39	100
	L	56.0	12.7	2.5	37	83
50-54	R	65.8	11.6	2.3	38	87
	L	57.3	10.7	2.1	35	76
55-59	R	57.3	12.5	2.5	33	86
	L	47.3	11.9	2.4	31	76
60-64	R	55.1	10.1	2.0	37	77
	L	45.7	10.1	2.0	29	66
65-69	R	49.6	9.7	1.8	35	74
	L	41.0	8.2	1.5	29	63
70-74	R	49.6	11.7	2.2	33	78
	L	41.5	10.2	1.9	23	67
75+	R	42.6	11.0	2.2	25	65
	L	37.6	8.9	1.7	24	61
All Female	R	62.8	17.0	.96	25	137
Subjects	L	53.9	15.7	.88	23	115

*The above mean scores for older subjects may be slightly low (0-10 pounds lower than they should be) due to instrument error detected after the study.

Reprinted with permission from the Archives of Physical Medicine and Rehabilitation, Volume 66, February 1985

Table 9

Average Performance of Normal Males on Key Pinch (pounds)

Age	Hand	Mean	SD	SE	Low	High
20-24	R	26.0	3.5	.65	21	34
	L	24.8	3.4	.64	19	31
25-29	R	26.7	4.9	.94	19	41
	L	25.0	4.4	.85	19	39
30-34	R	26.4	4.8	.93	20	36
	L	26.2	5.1	.98	17	36
35-39	R	26.1	3.2	.65	21	32
	L	25.6	3.9	.77	18	32
40-44	R	25.6	2.6	.50	21	31
	L	25.1	4.0	.79	19	31
45-49	R	25.8	3.9	.73	19	35
	L	24.8	4.4	.84	18	42
50-54	R	26.7	4.4	.88	20	34
	L	26.1	4.2	.84	20	37
55-59	R	24.2	4.2	.92	18	34
	L	23.0	4.7	1.02	13	31
60-64	R	23.2	5.4	1.13	14	37
	L	22.2	4.1	.84	16	33
65-69	R	23.4	3.9	.75	17	32
	L	22.0	3.6	.70	17	28
70-74	R	19.3	2.4	.47	16	25
	L	19.2	3.0	.59	13	28
75+	R	20.5	4.6	.1	9	31
	L	19.1	3.0	.59	13	24
All Male Subjects	R	24.5	4.6	.26	9	41
	L	23.6	4.6	.26	11	42

Reprinted with permission from the Archives of Physical Medicine and Rehabilitation, Volume 66, February 1985

Table 10

Average Performance of Normal Females on Key Pinch (pounds)

Age	Hand	Mean	SD	SE	Low	High
20-24	R	17.6	2.0	.39	14	23
	L	16.2	2.1	.41	13	23
25-29	R	17.7	2.1	.41	14	22
	L	16.6	2.1	.41	13	22
30-34	R	18.7	3.0	.60	13	25
	L	17.8	3.6	.70	12	26
35-39	R	16.6	2.0	.40	12	21
	L	16.0	2.7	.53	12	22
40-44	R	16.7	3.1	.56	10	24
	L	15.8	3.1	.55	8	22
45-49	R	17.6	3.2	.65	13	24
	L	16.6	2.9	.58	12	24
50-54	R	16.7	2.5	.50	12	22
	L	16.1	2.7	.53	12	22
55-59	R	15.7	2.5	.50	11	21
	L	14.7	2.2	.44	12	19
60-64	R	15.5	2.7	.55	10	20
	L	14.1	2.5	.50	10	19
65-69	R	15.0	2.6	.49	10	21
	L	14.3	2.8	.53	10	20
70-74	R	14.5	2.9	.54	8	22
	L	13.8	3.0	.56	9	22
75+	R	12.6	2.3	.45	8	17
	L	11.4	2.6	.50	7	16
All Female Subjects	R	16.2	3.0	.17	8	25
	L	15.3	3.1	.18	7	26

Reprinted with permission from the Archives of Physical Medicine and Rehabilitation, Volume 66, February 1985

TABLE 11

Average Performance of Normal Females on the Nine Hole Peg Test

(time in seconds)

Age	Hand	Mean	SD	SE	Low	High
20-24	R	15.8	2.1	.41	12	22
	L	17.2	2.4	.47	14	26
25-29	R	15.8	2.2	.43	13	23
	L	17.2	2.1	.40	15	25
30-34	R	16.3	1.9	.36	13	20
	L	17.8	2.0	.40	15	22
35-39	R	16.4	1.6	.32	14	20
	L	17.3	2.0	.40	15	21
40-44	R	16.8	2.1	.37	14	23
	L	18.6	2.8	.51	15	24
45-49	R	17.3	2.0	.39	13	23
	L	18.4	1.9	.38	16	24
50-54	R	18.0	2.5	.50	14	24
	L	20.1	3.0	.60	16	26
55-59	R	17.8	2.6	.52	14	26
	L	19.4	2.3	.47	16	24
60-64	R	18.4	2.0	.39	15	22
	L	20.6	2.2	.44	17	25
65-69	R	19.5	2.3	.44	16	25
	L	21.4	2.7	.51	17	26
70-74	R	20.2	2.7	.51	15	26
	L	22.0	2.7	.51	18	27
75+	R	21.5	2.9	.58	17	31
	L	24.6	4.3	.85	18	35
All Female Subjects	R	17.9	.8	.16	12	31
	L	19.6	3.4	.19	14	35

Reprinted with permission from the Archives of Physical Medicine and Rehabilitation, Volume 66, February 1985

TABLE 12

Average Performance of Normal Males on the Nine Hole Peg Test

(time in seconds)

Age	Hand	Mean	SD	SE	Low	High
20-24	R	16.1	1.9	.35	13	22
	L	16.8	2.2	.41	13	25
25-29	R	16.7	1.6	.31	15	21
	L	17.7	1.6	.31	15	21
30-34	R	17.7	2.5	.48	14	24
	L	18.7	2.2	.43	14	24
35-39	R	17.9	2.4	.48	15	26
	L	19.4	3.5	.70	14	28
40-44	R	17.7	2.2	.43	14	22
	L	18.9	2.0	.39	16	24
45-49	R	18.8	2.3	.43	15	24
	L	20.4	2.9	.55	15	27
50-54	R	19.2	1.8	.36	15	22
	L	20.7	2.3	.46	16	25
55-59	R	19.2	2.6	.56	14	25
	L	21.0	3.2	.70	17	27
60-64	R	20.3	2.6	.54	15	25
	L	21.0	2.5	.51	18	27
65-69	R	20.7	2.9	.55	15	29
	L	22.9	3.5	.67	18	30
70-74	R	22.0	3.3	.65	17	30
	L	28.8	3.9	.77	16	33
75+	R	22.9	4.0	.80	17	35
	L	26.4	4.8	.96	19	37
All Males Subjects	R	19.0	3.2	.18	13	35
	L	20.6	3.9	.22	13	37

Reprinted with permission from the Archives of Physical Medicine and Rehabilitation, Volume 66, February 1985

CHAPTER 4

USE OF THE PHYSICAL CAPACITIES EVALUATION IN THE REHABILITATION MODEL

THE CENTRAL COMPONENTS OF A WORK TOLER-ance program include adequate support from physicians, adequate space and equipment, careful planning, and the implementation of appropriate therapeutic activities and exercises. Then, a return-to-work phase completes the work tolerance services, and the physical capacities evaluation is used to determine each patient's ability to perform a job. Communication with the employer and insurance company representative is absolutely crucial to ensure smooth integration of the injured worker back into the workplace.

TEAM SUPPORT

The team members necessary to the success of a work tolerance program include administrators, physicians, nurses, physical and occupational therapists, and the patient. All efforts of the team must be directed toward returning the injured worker to work in a cost-effective, efficient amount of time. Administrators must realize the importance of a comprehensive therapy program. Physicians, also, must support the comprehensive services, including acute-care treatment as well as the work tolerance program.

Acute care is defined as the therapy services provided after trauma to stabilize the injured structures. Acute-care therapy includes wound care, support splinting to rest the injured part, splinting to prevent contractures, general active and passive range of motion exercises, instructions to the patient regarding edema control and exercises, and specialized evaluations for sensibility.

Work tolerance services include the provision of specific exercises to improve muscle strength, coordination, and endurance. Therapeutic activities are provided to improve the patient's functional capacity. Specific tasks are designed individually for each patient by the therapist to simulate the person's job requirements in a clinical setting.

The therapist tests the physical capacities in order to assess the patient's ability to perform regular job tasks. If the patient cannot perform enough of these tasks, the therapist makes specific recommendations for modifications and work capacity levels for the patient.

The philosophy and goals of the team must be united, so that the patient understands all the responsibilities connected with participating in the comprehensive program. The patient whose condition has improved to the subacute phase is required to attend therapy for progressively longer amounts of time in order to focus on improving strength and endurance. The physician must make the referral and explain to the patient the importance of attending therapy frequently, preferably three times weekly, for maximum benefit.

The patient must be closely monitored and guided through the work therapy rehabilitation program. The therapist must watch for use of substitution patterns and for avoidance of the use of the injured digit as a protective response. The patient must be aware that therapy is restricted to a definite time span and should participate in planning for his or her subsequent discharge. A study performed at the Hand Rehabilitation Center of Philadelphia in 1982 found that a patient participates in the work tolerance program an average of six weeks (Ballard et al. 1986).

Certain patients can easily resume normal activities and previous work tasks. However, patients who have severe injuries usually require a job change. Preparing for a job change should begin as soon as the patient's condition has plateaued and he or she is available for placement in a modified job. The therapist must communicate with the company's insurance carrier who assigns a rehabilitation specialist who assures that job placement is appropriate to the patient's physical abilities and restrictions.

SPACE, EQUIPMENT, AND SUPPLIES

Optimal space requirements for a work tolerance program are between 1,000 and 2,000 square feet. This amount of space is necessary because of the numerous physical tasks required of the patients. Someone lifting, carrying, pushing, or pulling an object requires walking space and space for assistive equipment, such as dollies. Adequate space assures that other patients will not be injured when a person is moving an object.

A work tolerance program can take place in a space as small as 200 square feet. However, in a restricted space, the therapist must be creative and use wall space and countertop space for multiple activities. A countertop can be used for woodworking, standardized tests, and ceramic hand molding; a wall space can be used for pulley exercises, lifting tasks, and therapeutic exercises.

In addition to the work tolerance space, other necessary areas include staff offices, waiting room reception area, secretarial offices, acute care therapy area, and, if possible, a separate work evaluation area. Acute-care therapy may need to be kept separated from the work tolerance program if therapeutic activities would contaminate open wounds. Sanding, painting, staining, or woodworking projects should not occur where open wounds are debrided and dressed. The work tolerance area should have ventilation that is adequate for exhausting the dust and fumes produced by therapeutic activities.

All areas of the work tolerance program must have a staff member present when patients are performing exercises and activities. In particular, no room should be left unsupervised while patients are performing resistive exercises.

The blueprints of the Hand Rehabilitation Services of Atlanta indicate excellent use of all available space (Figures 1,2). The blueprints illustrate the creative use of space for clinical treatment.

Since equipment and supplies require a significant amount of space, clinics may expand as the patient population grows (Figures 3,4).

Equipment for a work tolerance program includes evaluation equipment, therapeutic activity equipment, job simulation equipment, modalities, and office equipment. Equipment should be durable and designed to withstand heavy clinical use.

Therapeutic exercisers should be purchased for general body conditioning, as well as for specific upper extremity conditioning. Selection of standardized tests should be based on occupations prevalent in the geographical area of the clinical setting. The therapist may wish to limit the initial purchase of standardized tests until patients' occupations can be analyzed. Otherwise, say, if an electrical circuitry work sample is purchased, and the patients in the area perform assembly line jobs and machine operation jobs, the standardized tests will have little applicability.

Selection of therapeutic activities and equipment is based on the space available, staff available for craft instructions, and the beneficial effect of the craft activity on the population treated, and the physical demands of the occupations that are prevalent in the area. For example, wood carving is an appropriate therapeutic activity for a population of laborers or carpenters, but not for electronic assemblers.

Evaluation equipment suggested in the work tolerance program includes the following:

Evaluation Equipment/Resource Company

Boley gauge
North Coast Medical, Inc.
187 Stauffer Blvd.
San Jose, CA 95125

Bags of gravel (including 10-, 25-, 35-, 50-, and 100-lb. bags)
Local garden supply store

Box with dowel and slotted handles
Fabricated by Tim Powers based on
Kenneth Blankenship's design (Figure 5)

Box with side handles
Fabricated by Tim Powers, designed by Susan Smith,
M.S., OTR (Figure 6)

BTE work simulator (lease plan)
Baltimore Therapeutic Equipment Co.
7455-L New Ridge Road
Hanover, MD 21076-3105

Disk weights, one set, and Dumbbells, two sets with 1–25 lb. weights
Local sporting goods store or
J.A. Preston Corporation
60 Page Road
Clifton, NJ 07012

Finger circumference gauge
Fred Sammons, Inc.
Box 32
Brookfield, IL 60413-0032

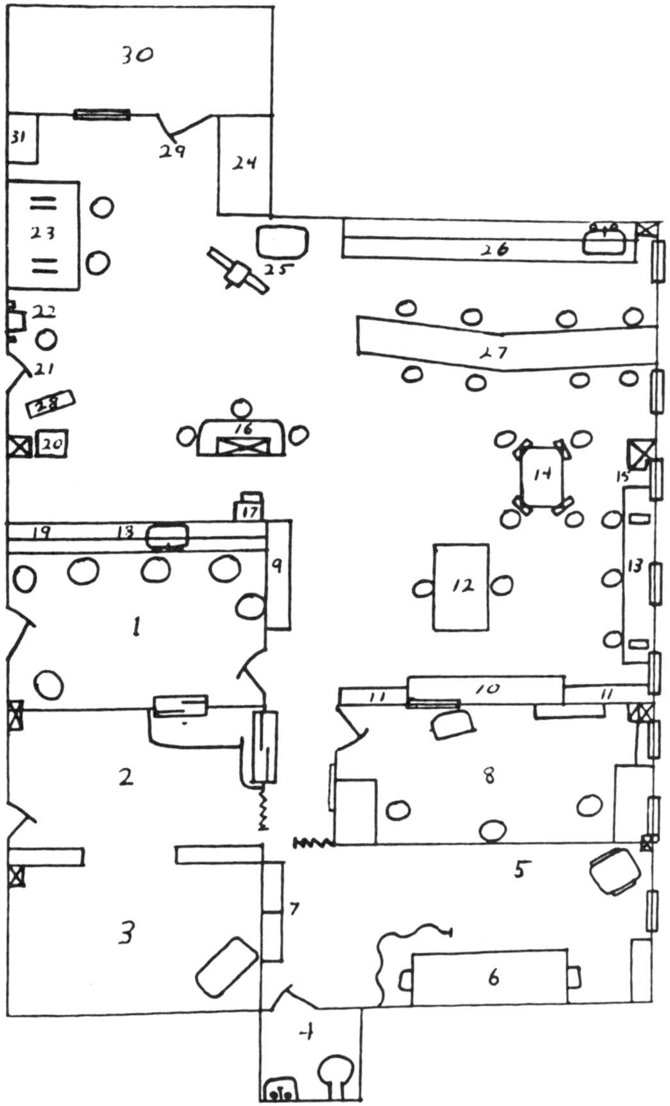

HAND REHABILITATION CENTER OF ATLANTA, INC.

LAYOUT OF CLINIC

OFFICE AREAS

1. Waiting room and reception area.
2. Office Manager, Administration
3. Secretarial and transcription, copy machine, patient files and storage for office supplies
4. Bathroom
8. Office for Director of Center and Clinical Director
30. Therapists' office

ONE-ON-ONE AREA

5. Relaxation and biofeedback
6. Curtained off area for specific upper extremity problems, such as scapula and shoulder.
7. Clinic library

MAIN CLINIC

9. Storage, refreshments, hydrauculator and paraffin
10. Moderate and work oriented activities
11. Light activities as well as desensitization
12. Desensitization as well as area for specific activities (elevated table)
13. Elevation boards for edema as well as macrame area and one-on-one area as well as light activities
14. Progressive resistive exercises (weight wells and pinch & pulls)
15. Home, work and leisure tools (fishing pole, rifle, rakes, shovel, etc.)
16. Leather area
17. Volumetric measurements
18. Whirlpool, debridement and wound care
19. Specific physical modalities
20. Refrigerator
21. Shoulder pulleys and walk up ladder
22. Super II (resistive body exercisor)
23. Sanding table
24. Woodworking and storage for stimulators
25. B.T.E. (Work evaluator)
26. Supplies, splint fabrication
27. Evaluation and documentation as well as education and one-on-one
28. Fluidotherapy
29. Over door pulleys
31. Light to moderate activities storage

Reprinted with permission from the Hand Rehabilitation Center, Inc., Atlanta, GA.

Figure 2 The layout in Figure 1 is identified by the numbered key.

Reprinted with permission from the Hand Rehabilitation Center, Inc., Atlanta, GA.

Figure 1 Hand Rehabilitation Center of Atlanta initially provided comprehensive services in 1,000 square feet of clinic space.

The Hand Rehabilitation Center of Atlanta, Inc., consists of two clinics and a third satellite clinic. All activities and devices are kept in view of the patients (pegboards/shelves) and not stored.

AREAS

1. Combination library/kitchen
2. Center Director's office
3. Clinical Director and one staff therapist's office
4. Staff therapists' office
5. Staff restroom
6,7,8 & 10. Business office; office manager, transcriptionist, receptionist, patient files, computer and data collection. Patients check in at the window between 9 and 10 and schedule next appointments in front of receptionist desk at 10.
9. Patient waiting room with electronic locking door to clinic (this keeps people from coming into the clinic unwanted)
11. Biofeedback/relaxation
12. Shoulder room. Waist high table with mat, hydrocollator, ultrasound and electrical stimulation cart, wall desk
13. Observation/quiet room. One way mirrors for observing into main clinic, telephone for talking to M.D.'s, etc., and x-ray viewer. Walls are double insulated
14. Shoulder ladder
15. Overhead whirlpool
16. Elevated hydrotherapy and wound care
17. Volumetric testing
18. Desensitization/sensory re-education (elevated table)
19. Paraffin/dynamic splinting treatment
20. Hot packs, towels/storage
21. Exercise, edema control, shoulder work, one on one (elevated table with storage underneath)
22. Light resistive exercise devices
23. Refreshment area (coffee, tea, water)
(24-33). (Advanced work hardening area)
24. Work related activities
25. Super II - resistive body exerciser
26. Shoulder pulleys
27. Storage/evaluation/one on one
28. Work related activities and timed testing/one on one
29. Macrame
30. Light activities/crafts/free weights
31. Work related activities/Valpar/small engine break down, other timed tests
32. B.T.E.
33. Evaluation/one on one
34. Leather crafts
35. Progressive resistive weight training
36. Evaluation/splint fabrication/ one on one
37. Splinting area
38. Evaluation/storage carousel/refrigerator/relaxation area
39. Small activities/one on one/typing, adding machines, etc. (table has built-in elevation stations).
40-43. Woodworking area (this area is enclosed with glass so it can be viewed from all directions and still maintain sound/dust control.
40. Wood project storage
41. Work bench/hand tools
42. Elevated progressive resistive, sanding
43. Flat sanding/carving/project completion area
44. Fluidotherapy

Reprinted with permission from the Hand Rehabilitation Center, Ltd., Atlanta, GA.

Figure 4 Areas in Figure 3 are identified by the numbered key.

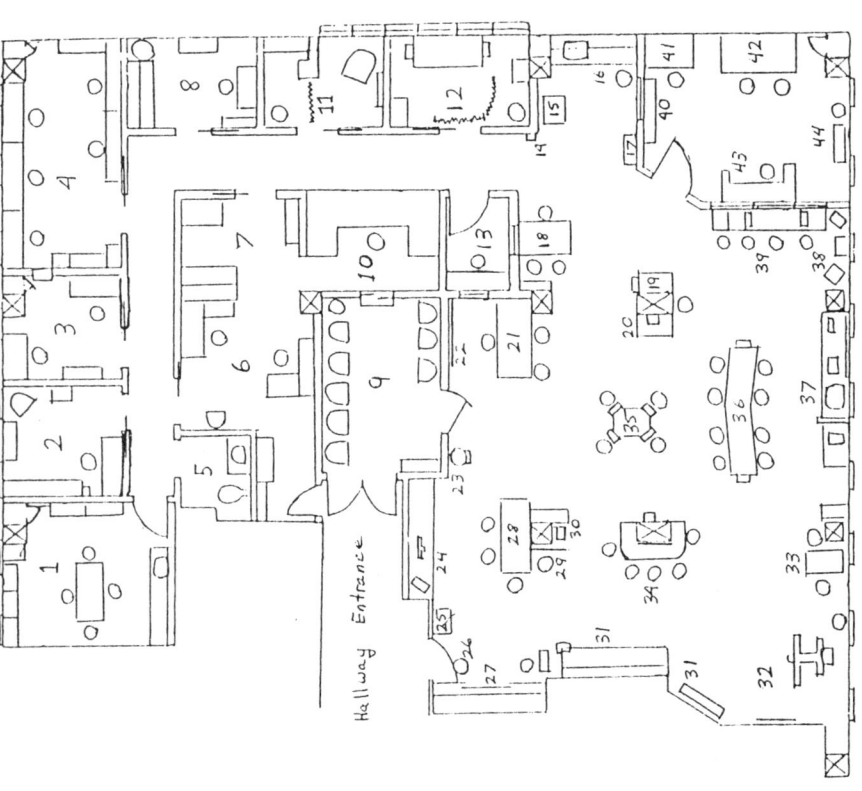

~~~ : Curtains

OΠ : Chairs

: Wooden pocket doors; open into the wall; space saver

: Cabinet with cupboard above

Reprinted with permission from the Hand Rehabilitation Center, Inc., Atlanta, GA.

Figure 3 The work tolerance area of the Hand Rehabilitation Center of Atlanta are integrated into the patient care area.

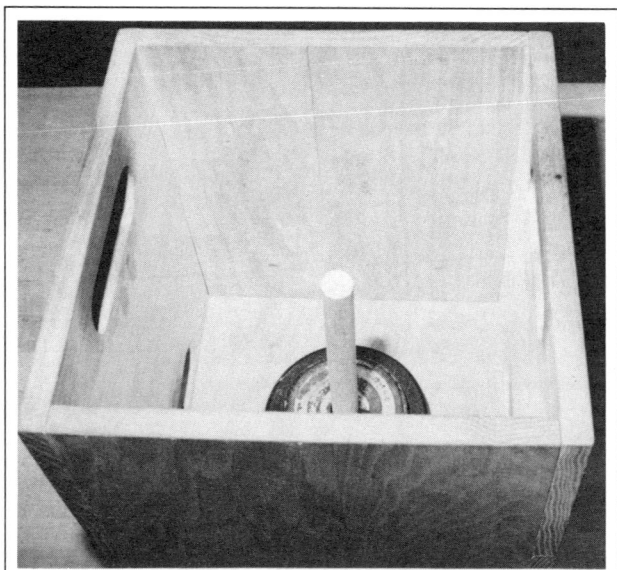

Reprinted with permission from the Hand Rehabilitation Center, Ltd., Philadelphia, PA.

Figure 5 This box is used if the weight needs to be stabilized on the dowel.

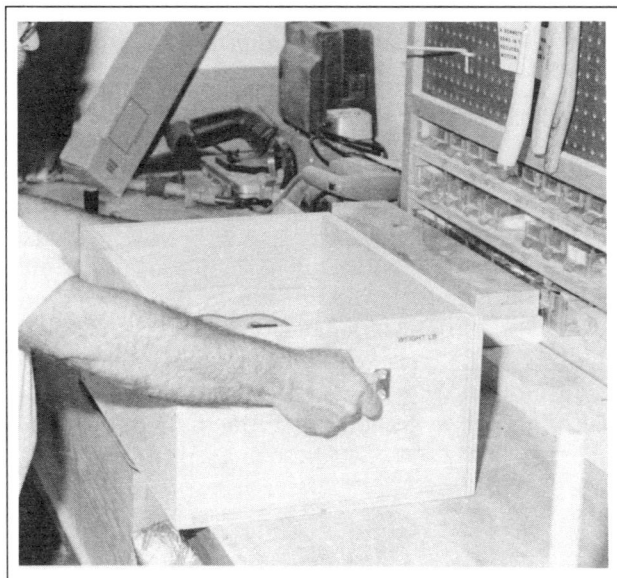

Reprinted with permission from the Hand Rehabilitation Center, Ltd., Philadelphia, PA.

Figure 6 This box, designed by Smith, is easy for patients to lift due to handles on each side.

Goniometers (order for shoulder, elbow, and wrist)
J.A. Preston Corporation
60 Page Road
Clifton, NJ 07012

Goniometer for finger
Fred Sammons, Inc.

Hand Volumeter
Volumeters Unlimited
52421 Double View Drive
P.O. Box 146
Idlewild, CA 92347

Industrial buckets
Local hardware store

Jebsen-Taylor Hand Function test
Fabricated by staff; reference: *Archives of Physical Medicine and Rehabilitation*, June 1969, pp. 311–19.

Milk crates
Local general store

Minnesota Rate of Manipulation test
J.A. Preston Corporation

Moberg Pick-Up test
Volumeters, Unlimited

Pipe Assembly
Fabricated by Debbie Beaulieu, OTR, and Tim Powers. Pipes available in local plumbing store (Figure 7)

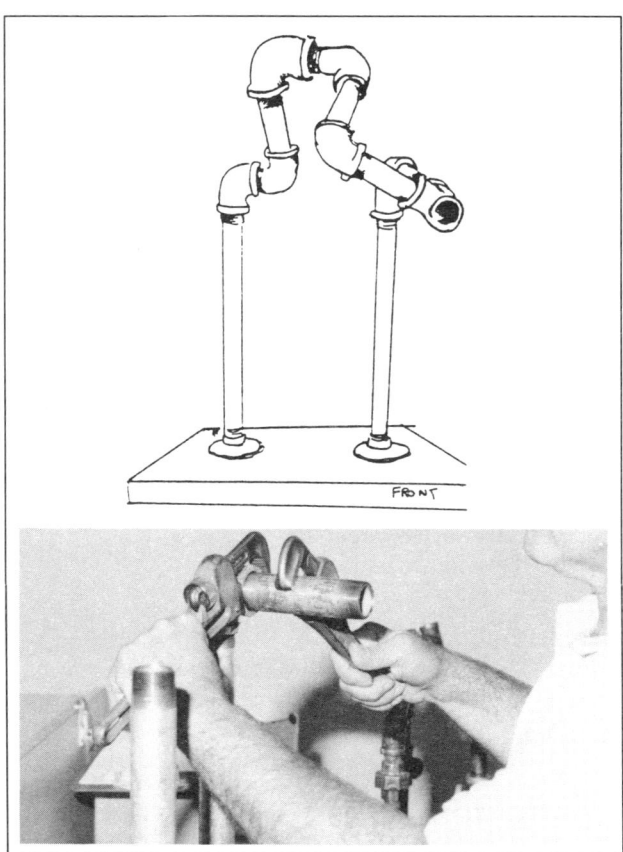

Reprinted with permission from the Hand Rehabilitation Center, Ltd., Philadelphia, PA.

Figure 7 Construction of the pipe assembly enables a patient to work with wrenches bilaterally.

Powers lifting frame
Fabricated by Tim Powers (Figure 8)

Pinch gauge
J.A. Preston Corporation

Semmes-Weinstein monofilaments
Volumeters, Unlimited

Purdue Pegboard test
J.A. Preston Corporation

Stopwatch
Local sporting goods store

Valpar Work Samples: Small Tools Mechanical Work Sample, Upper Extremity Range of Motion Work Sample, Whole Body Range of Motion Work Sample, Simulated Assembly Work Sample
Valpar Corporation
P.O. Box 5767
Tucson, AZ 85703-5767

Equipment for Therapeutic Activities/ Resource Company

Adaptive ADL equipment
Fred Sammons, Inc., and
Susquehanna Rehab, RD2
9 Overlook Drive
Wrightsville, PA

Bilateral sanders
Designed and fabricated by Tim Powers (Figure 9); also available through Fred Sammons, Inc.

Ceramic potter's wheel
NASCO Arts & Crafts
901 Janesville Avenue
Fort Atkinson, WI 53538

Ceramic tool set
NASCO Arts & Crafts

Concept II Rowing Ergometer
Concept II Inc.
RR1 Box 1100
Morrisville, VT 05661-9727

Cybex Extremity System 350
Cybex Division of Lumex Inc.
Ronkonkoma, NY 11779

Desensitization kit
Fabricated by Joanne DiMattia. Includes lambswool, nylon, burlap, and denim materials.

Door latch frame kit
J.A. Preston Corporation

Dressing frames
Sensory re-education kit, including tactile textures set; tactile numbers set
J.A. Preston Corporation
Dumbbells, 2 sets 1–25 lb.
Local sporting goods store or J.A. Preston

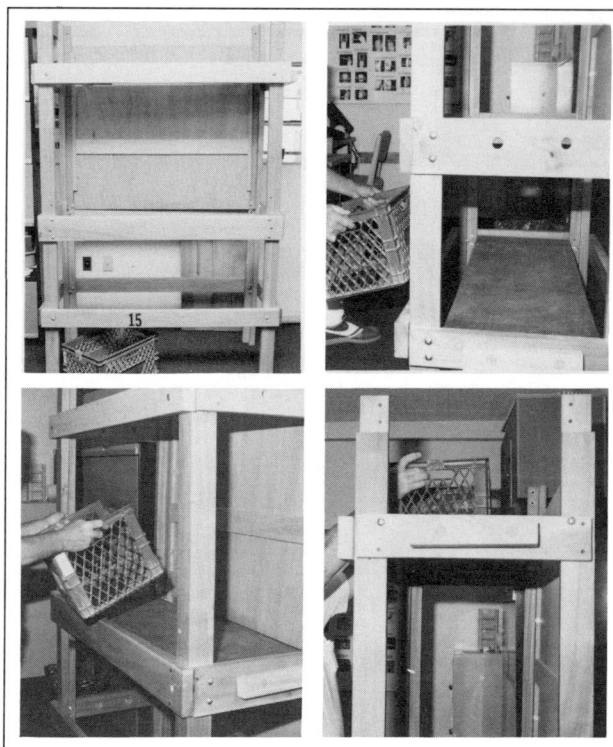

Reprinted with permission from the Hand Rehabilitation Center, Ltd., Philadelphia, PA.

Figure 8 The lifting frame enables the therapist to observe the patient lifting at various heights.

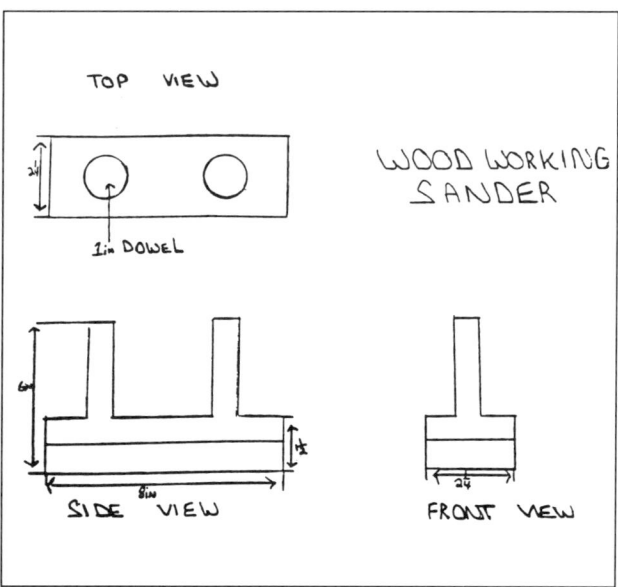

Reprinted with permission from the Hand Rehabilitation Center, Ltd., Philadelphia, PA.

Figure 9 The bilateral sander is used during woodworking and during exercises.

Elevation board
Designed by Gisela Hall (Figure 10)

Exercycle
J.A. Preston Corporation

Extension board exerciser
Fabricated by Tim Powers (Figure 11)

Hydra Fitness
Hydra Gym Athletics Inc.
P.O. Box 599-2121
Industrial Park Road
Belton, TX 76513

Kiln
NASCO Arts & Crafts

Leathercraft tool set
Tandy's Leather
122 S. 12th Street
Philadelphia, PA 19107

Macrame cord, beads, and rings
Vanguard Crafts
17101 Utica Avenue
Brooklyn, NY 11234

Macrame hanger
Fabricated by Tim Powers, (Figure 12)

Nordic Track
141 Jonathan Blvd.
North Chaska, MN 55318

Prehension pegboard
J.A. Preston Corporation

Prehension Pegboard
J.A. Preston, Corporation

Rowing machine
Concept II, Inc.
RD1, Box 1100
Morrisville, VT 05661

Stair Master 4000 P.T.
Randal Sports Medical Products
12421 Willows Road
Northeast Suite 100
Kirkland, WA 98034

UBE Ergometer
Cybex Metabolic Systems
Cybex Division of Lumex Inc.
Ronkonkoma, NY 11779

Wall pulley
J.A. Preston Corporation

Weight rack
Fabricated by Tim Powers (Figure 13)

Woodworking tool set
J.A. Preston Corporation

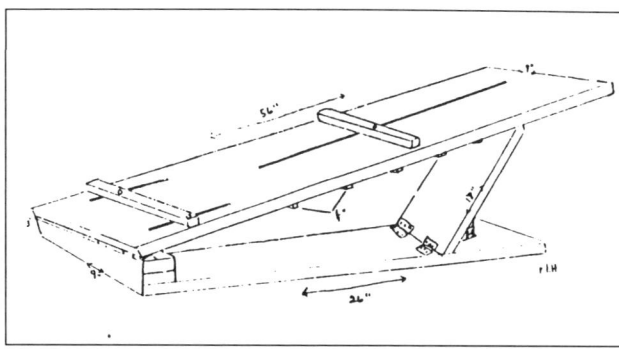

Reprinted with permission from the Hand Rehabilitation Center, Ltd., Philadelphia, PA.

Figure 10 Resistive shoulder flexion exercises are performed on the elevation board.

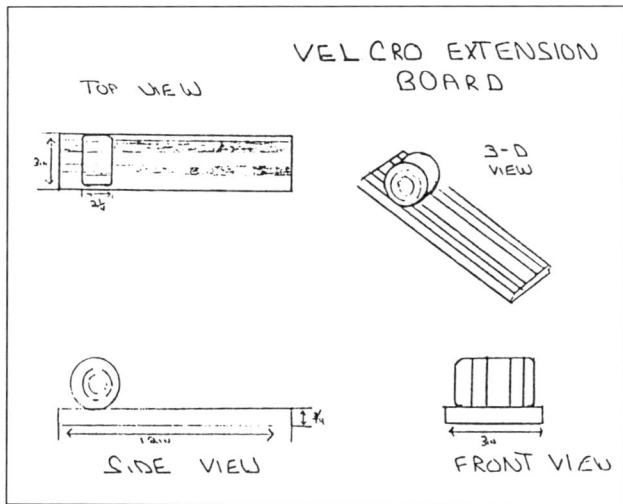

Reprinted with permission from the Hand Rehabilitation Center, Ltd., Philadelphia, PA.

Figure 11 Resisted digit extension exercises are performed by using the extension board.

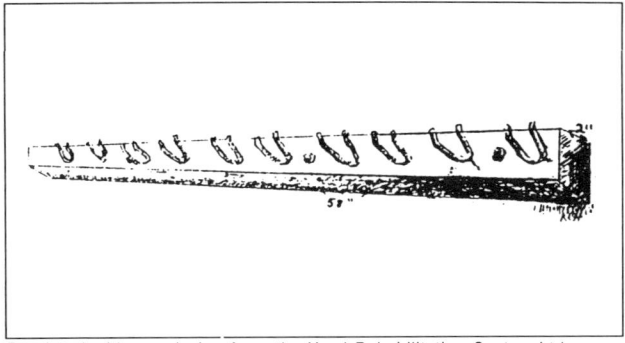

Reprinted with permission from the Hand Rehabilitation Center, Ltd., Philadelphia, PA.

Figure 12 This macrame hanger assists in working on a macrame project with hands elevated above the heart, which reduces swelling of the hands.

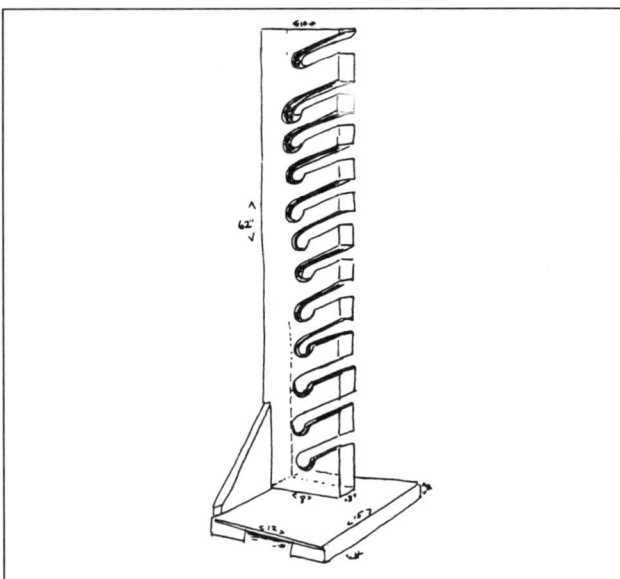

Reprinted with permission from the Hand Rehabilitation Center, Ltd., Philadelphia, PA.

Figure 13 The weight rack stores dumbbells in an organized, accessible frame.

Wood carving tool set
J.A. Preston Corporation

Woodworking benches
SATCO
924 S. 19th Avenue
Minneapolis, MN 55404

Modalities for Therapy/Resource Company

Arm whirlpool
J.A. Preston Corporation

Electrical stimulation machine
Cleo, Inc.
3975 Mayfield Road
Cleveland, OH 44121

Fluidotherapy
Henley International
104 Industrial Blvd.
Sugarland, TX 77478

Hot-pack machine
J.A. Preston Corporation

Parrafin bath
J.A. Preston Corporation

Ultrasound Unit
Cleo, Inc.

Verimed computerized biofeedback
Verimed Company, Inc.
1401 E. Broward Blvd.
or 10001 N.W. 62nd St.
Fort Lauderdale, FL 33339

Vibrator, small
Lillian Vernon
Susquehanna Rehab
9 Overlook Drive
Wrightsville, PA 17368

JOB SIMULATION EQUIPMENT

Bags
Local garden supply store

Boxes

Dumbbells and disc weights (Figure 14)
J.A. Preston Corporation

Lifting Frame
(Figure 8)

Pipe assembly
(Figure 7)

Valpar Work Samples
Valpar Corporation

Work simulator
Baltimore Therapeutic Equipment Co.

STAFFING THE WORK TOLERANCE PROGRAM

Often, there is not enough staff to provide the multiple services required in a work tolerance program. In order to contain costs, therapists perform evaluations, plan treatment, and supervise staff and patients. Aides teach therapeutic activities and assist patients according to the orders of the doctors and therapists. Art instructors and woodworking instructors closely supervise patients during therapeutic activities.

Therapists design all job simulation tasks on the basis of the patient's actual job requirements. They perform all evaluations as well, including initial evaluations, progress evaluations, physical capacities evaluations, and activities of daily living evaluations. Therapists also provide written home programs for desensitization, resistive exercises, therapeutic activities, activities of daily living, and protection of joints.

REFERRALS

Referrals may come from physicians, rehabilitation nurses, insurance companies, and the patients themselves. In some states, therapists can evaluate patients without a doctor's referral. In other states, a doctor's referral is required by law. To maximize the referral base, therapists should speak at professional conferences and publish articles in order to disseminate information about the services provided in the work tolerance program.

When physicians refer patients to the work tolerance program, they identify the patient's level of resistance. There are five levels of resistance based on the amount of weight the patient can use during performance of therapeutic exercises:

Level I: 0-1 pound of resistance during coordination training, prehension activities, desensitization, and therapeutic activities involving elevation to reduce edema

Level II: 1-3 pounds of resistance during therapeutic exercises and the therapeutic activities of leatherwork, ceramics, and woodworking

Level III: 3-30 pounds of resistance during therapeutic exercises and therapeutic activities, including woodworking, ceramic molding on the potter's wheel, use of the work simulator, and specific job-simulated tasks

Level IV: 30-60 pounds of resistance during therapeutic exercises and therapeutic activities, including wood carving and specific job-simulated tasks

Level V: 60-150 pounds of resistance during therapeutic exercises and job simulation.

Physicians are instructed to refer patients according to the level of resistance specific injured structures can tolerate. Physicians have a high level of understanding of this concept and make referrals based on the patients' levels of resistance. Patients should start no higher than level III, in order to minimize muscle discomfort following the performance of the therapeutic exercises. Patients may be referred for level I and advanced according to the therapist's evaluation together with results of regular communication between the physician and therapist.

PLANNING THE WORK TOLERANCE PROGRAM

In order to plan an appropriate work tolerance program, data must be gathered concerning the patient's diagnosis, extent of injury, and job requirements and the physician's orders for rehabilitation services. During the initial referral, the therapist should discuss with the physician the operative procedure, the integrity of the injured structures such as tendons, nerves, and fractured bones, the projected length of treatment, and the prognosis.

In order to plan effective treatment, the therapist should evaluate the condition of the patient's upper extremity. Therapists are encouraged to use a problem-solving reporting format to structure their plans for therapy. If short-term goals are set and accomplished, treatment will be effective. Initially, a pa-

tient's swelling and pain may respond quickly to elevated prehension tasks and appropriate modalities. Later, in the subacute phase, the patient's problems may be stiffness of joints and limited strength. Stiffness of joints is treated through the use of therapeutic modalities, splinting, and a program to strengthen muscles. Muscle strength is improved through therapeutic exercises and therapeutic activities. As muscle strength improves, the patient is able to achieve the maximum tendon excursion needed to increase joint motion. Final goals of therapy focus on the patient's ability to use the injured upper extremity for functional work and avocational activities.

Treatment goals focus on specific job requirements. To obtain information concerning the patient's job, the *Dictionary of Occupational Titles* (U.S. Dept. of Labor, 1991; hereafter *DOT*) can be used. This reference work includes descriptions for several thousand jobs. The therapist may obtain a job analysis from a rehabilitation nurse or the personnel manager in the patient's work organization. In addition, the therapist may arrange an on-site visit early in the patient's program so that appropriate job simulation can be designed in the clinic.

The Dictionary of Occupational Titles (U.S. Dept.of Labor, 1991) is used to obtain information about the physical demands, environmental conditions and specific vocational preparation required for each job listed in the *DOT*. In using the reference, the therapist should gather information in the following manner:

1) Refer to the alphabetical index of job titles starting on page 1225 in Volume II of the *Dictionary of Occupational Titles*. For example, look under "T" for truck driver and obtain the *DOT* code # (for truck driver, heavy, which is 905.663-014).

2) There are two volumes of the *Dictionary of Occupational Titles*. Volume I includes jobs with *DOT* codes from 00/01 through 599.687–038. For the truck driver job description you would look in Volume II for the *DOT* code 905.663-014. Review the job description to define physical demands of the job.

3) After the specific job description is located, look at the definition trailer for the strength rating.

4) Refer to page 1012 for the level of work and strength rating indicated in the definition trailer for heavy truck driver. The strength factor pertains to the amount of weight that must be lifted, carried, pushed, or pulled on the job. Medium work is defined as occasional lifting

of up to 50 pounds with frequent lifting and carrying of up to 25 pounds.

5) Look on page XVII for the definition of the various parts of the definition trailer.

A description of the patient's job demands can be developed through an occupational interview with the patient during the initial evaluation. The patient's opinion is obtained on the physical demands of the job and the specific job duties. The patient is asked to estimate the amount of lifting and carrying required, including the maximum and the average amount of weight, the frequency of lifting, the range of lifting, and the types of objects lifted. Pushing and pulling are also examined, and the maximum amount of weight, the height involved, the average amount of weight, the frequency involved, and whether any assistive devices are used in pushing and pulling are ascertained.

For an analysis of reaching, the patient is asked the ranges in which lifting is required. Each range is broken down into floor level, knee level, waist level, shoulder level, and above shoulder level, and the appropriate ones are identified. The patient describes the types of objects he or she handles and manipulates, and identifies specific hand and power tools.

Additional job tasks, such as climbing, kneeling, crouching, crawling, standing, and walking, are analyzed by the patient. The occupational interview also reviews the patient's functional status and medical precautions, as well as the need for a formal job analysis and on-site visit (Figure 15).

A form letter and job analysis form are sent to the personnel manager or the rehabilitation specialist assigned to manage the patient's case, usually, the former (Figure 16). The letter points out that the information will be used to design the therapy program and evaluation of the patient's physical capacities. The physical demands of the job are listed, and the personnel manager fills in the details based on observation and description of the job.

Lifting, carrying, pushing, and pulling are physical demands requiring specific identification of the weight used for each and the frequency of performing the tasks. The range of reaching is outlined, and manipulation and tool handling are noted in detail. The tools used, as well as the additional physical demands performed on the job, are also noted. The working environment and the possible job arrangements in the company are also considered.

If the therapist needs additional information to plan the patient's evaluation and treatment, an on-site job evaluation is necessary. The financial arrangements

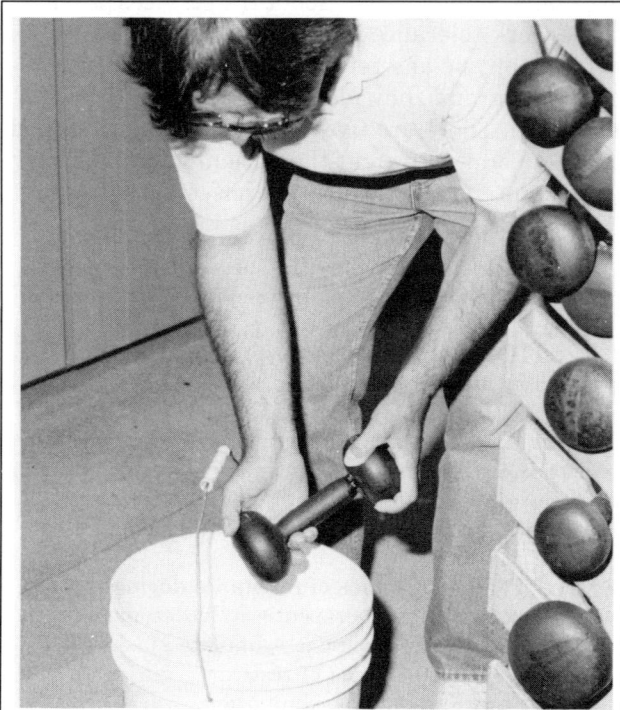

Reprinted with permission from the Hand Rehabilitation Center, Ltd., Philadelphia, PA.

Figure 14 Patients perform repetitive lifting by placing dumbbells in an industrial bucket.

must be approved by the insurance company in advance. The insurance claims adjuster is informed of the need for the therapist to visit the plant to observe the job performance closely (Figure 17).

After approval has been obtained, the insurance claims adjuster sets a time for the therapist to visit with the personnel manager. The therapist should dress appropriately for walking and standing in all types of industrial conditions. Flat, sturdy shoes are appropriate and a laboratory coat or uniform is recommended in order to identify the therapist as one of the medical personnel. A business suit may also be worn; however, employers may then confuse the therapist with someone from the business or the insurance company.

The therapist should perform the on-site job evaluation by observing an employee performing the patient's job. Again, the amount of weight lifted, carried, pushed, or pulled is noted, as are the frequency and range of lifting and carrying, etc. Reaching, manipulating, and the performance of other job tasks are recorded, as are the type of working environment and the tools used. The therapist may discuss with the employer the possibility of the patient's returning to part-time work, full-time work, or modified

OCCUPATIONAL INTERVIEW

Name: _____ Initial Treatment Date: _____

Age: _____ Dominant Hand: Right: _____ Left: _____

Phone: _____ Injured Hand: Right: _____ Left: _____

Injury: _____

Diagnosis: _____

Additional Medical Problems: _____

Occupation: _____

REQUIREMENTS OF JOB:

LIFTING:

Frequency: _____ Average Amount: _____ Maximum Amount: _____

Plane of Lifting: _____ Types of Objects: _____

CARRYING:

Frequency: _____ Average Amount: _____ Maximum Amount: _____

Plane of Carrying: _____ Types of Objects: _____

PUSHING/PULLING:

Types of Objects: _____ Weight of Objects: _____

Assistive Devices Used: _____ Frequency: _____

REACHING:

Planes of Reaching: _____ Frequency: _____

Types of Objects: _____

HANDLING:

Types of Objects: _____ Weight of Objects: Maximum _____
Average _____

MANIPULATING:

Types of Objects: _____ Frequency: _____

Speed Required: _____ Tools Used: _____

Additional Physical Demands: _____

Request Job Analysis: _____ Request On-Site Visit: _____

Reprinted with permission from the Hand Rehabilitation Center, Ltd., Philadelphia, PA.

Figure 15 An occupational interview is used to collect data from the patient during the initial visit.

HAND REHABILITATION CENTER LTD.

901 WALNUT STREET
PHILA., PA. 19107
Telephone (215) 629-0980

Surgery:
James M. Hunter, M.D.
Lawrence H. Schneider, M.D.
Scott H. Jaeger, M.D.
Marwan A. Wehbé, M.D.
Stephen L. Cash, M.D.

Hand Therapy:
Evelyn J. McKim, L.P.T., Director
Anne D. Callahan, M.S., O.T.R./L, Asst. Director
Patricia L. Baxter, O.T.R./L
Pamela McEntee, O.T.R./L
Wandra Miles, O.T.R./L
Melanie Ballard, O.T.R./L
Richard Read, R.P.T.
Barbara Goodwin, R.P.T.
Paula Bremm-Keder, R.P.T.
Susan Toth, O.T.R./L
Patricia M. Byron, M.A., O.T.R.
Elaine Muntzer, R.P.T.
Laura A. Bruening, O.T.R./L
Susan Tribuzi, O.T.R./L
Marianne Koehler, O.T.R./L
Karen M. Stewart, M.S., O.T.R./L

Administrator
Charles W. Coombs   JOB DESCRIPTION AND JOB ANALYSIS

Dear Employer:

To facilitate treatment of _____ we request information concerning the job requirements this person performed. Please fill in the information as detailed as possible.

Job Description: _____

Physical Demands of Job: 1) Lifting: maximum amount: _____

Repetition of lifting maximum amount: _____

Average amount of weight lifted: _____

Frequency of lifting average amount of weight: _____

Types of objects lifted in work: _____

2) Objects carried at work: _____

Frequency of carrying objects at work: _____

Types of adaptive equipment utilized for carrying objects (hand truck): _____

Reprinted with permission from the Hand Rehabilitation Center, Ltd., Philadelphia, PA.

Figure 16 A form letter is sent to the patient's personnel manager requesting a completed job analysis form. The personnel manager describes the physical demands of the job by completing the job description and job analysis form.

61

Figure 16 (Continued)

3) Pushing/pulling: types of objects pushed and pulled: _____

Assistive equipment utilized for pushing and pulling: _____

4) Reaching: a) above shoulder level _____

b) below waist level _____

5) Walking, standing, sitting: _____

6) Handling: types of objects handled: _____

7) Frequency of gross handling as is required to stabilize an object: _____

8) Frequency of pick-up, grasp, release-type of handling: _____

9) Manipulating: types of objects manipulated: _____

Amount of rapid manipulation required: _____

10) Climbing/balancing: climbing ladders: _____

climbing stairs: _____ balancing while climbing: _____

Is gripping required for safety during climbing? YES _____ NO _____ .

11) Feeling: does employee handle objects in environments outside or in cold or hot environments? YES _____ NO _____ .

12) Endurance: Is heavy repetitive lifting, carrying, pushing, and pulling required for prolonged periods of time? YES _____ NO _____

13) Is employee required to work in hazardous situations? YES _____ NO _____

Please explain. _____

Are job modifications allowed? Yes/No

If yes, describe: _____

Is part-time work available? Yes/No

If yes, describe: _____

Thank you for your assistance!

When completed, please return to:

Hand Rehabilitation Center, LTD.
ATTN: _____
901 Walnut Street
Philadelphia, PA 19107

Reprinted with permission from the Hand Rehabilitation Center, Ltd., Philadelphia, PA.

Figure 16 *Continued*

HAND REHABILITATION CENTER, LTD.

901 WALNUT STREET
PHILA, PA 19107
Telephone (215) 629-0980

Surgery:
James M. Hunter, M.D.
Lawrence H. Schneider, M.D.
Scott H. Jaeger, M.D.
Stephen J. Cash, M.D.

Administrator of Rehabilitation
Evelyn J. Mackin, L.P.T.

Hand Therapy Staff:
Paula Breme Kader, R.P.T.
Patricia L. Baxter, O.T.R/L
Anne D. Callahan, M.S., O.T.R./L.
Richard Reed, R.P.T.
Susan Toth, O.T.R./L.
Patricia M. Byron, MA., O.T.R./L.
Laura A. Bruening, O.T.R./L.
Susan Tribuzi, O.T.R./L.
Marianne Koehler, O.T.R./L.
Karen M. Stewart, MS., O.T.R./L.
Frank Angiolillo, R.P.T.
Gwendolyn van Strien, R.P.T.
Gisele Larose, O.T.R./L.
Susan Blackmore, O.T.R./L
Barbara L. Reeder, O.T.R./L
Debra Beaulieu, O.T.R./L.
Colleen Burke, P.T.A.

TO: _____

FROM: _____

RE: _____
Claim # _____
HRC# _____

Dear _____

We are requesting permission for an on-site visit to assess _____'s job. The purpose of this visit is to enable the therapist to learn more about the patient's job. This process will facilitate treatment and discharge planning specific to the patient's job to enable _____ (him or her) to return to work as soon as possible.

This visit will take _____ hours and the fee will be approximately _____. The travel fee will be approximately _____

Your prompt consideration in this matter is appreciated. Thank you.

Sincerely,

_____

When completed, please return to the Hand Rehabilitation Center, Ltd.,
ATTN: _____ 901 Walnut Street, Philadelphia,
Pennsylvania, 19107.

Reprinted with permission from the Hand Rehabilitation Center, Ltd., Philadelphia, PA.

Figure 17 A form letter goes to the patient's insurance claims adjuster to obtain financial approval for an on-site visit.

work. Allowances for use of splints, adaptive equipment, and a modified work arrangement are considered, if necessary (Figure 18).

TREATMENT

Therapeutic exercises, therapeutic activities, and job simulation tasks are chosen on the basis of the patient's particular physical injury and job requirements. Ten exercises and five activities are used regularly. Each patient's program is individually designed based on tolerance, strength, and endurance. The patient is closely monitored to ensure that the program is not causing increased swelling or pain.

Strength, hand volume, range of motion, coordination, and endurance are evaluated regularly. Hand volume is recorded before and after each therapy session if swelling is a problem. Grip and pinch strength are recorded once a week. Coordination is evaluated once every three to four weeks in order to allow for sufficient improvement prior to subsequent testing. Endurance is tested weekly, using the BTE work simulator.

THERAPEUTIC EXERCISE

The therapeutic exercises used in the work tolerance program include isometric exercises, isotonic exercises, and isokinetic exercises. Isometric exercises are used initially for any patient who has pain or is restricted from repetitive resistive motions. Isometric exercise is a sustained contraction of the muscle in one position (Gimby et al. 1973). Isometrics can be performed by having the patient contract and hold the contraction of any major muscle group for five seconds and then repeat 20 times, twice a day. The Verimed biofeedback unit is used to increase isometric muscle contractions. The patient views a screen that indicates the motor action potential of the muscles. The biofeedback unit can be used with dual channels to encourage the patient to relax the antagonist muscles while attempting to increase muscle contraction of the agonist muscle. The work simulator can also be used for isometric muscle contraction routines. The device is set to the static manual mode, and the patient contracts the muscles while applying force against each tool that does not move.

Isotonic exercises are used after the initial acute phase of treatment as the patient gains strength. Isotonic exercises are dynamic muscle contractions against resistance without control of the speed of movement (Zinovieff 1951). Progressive resistive exercises are performed with free weights to facilitate

rapid strengthening of the extrinsic muscle groups (Figure 19).

A 1980 study at the Hand Rehabilitation Center of Philadelphia, Ltd., correlated the amount of weight a patient could lift during a stress test with grip strength. The results yielded the following ranges:

Grip Measurements	Lifting Ability
5–10 lb.	1–3 lb.
10–20 lb.	3–5 lb.
20–30 lb.	5–7 lb.
30–60 lb.	8–10 lb.
60 lb. or more	10–12 lb.

This scale is used instead of a stress test to reduce the initial set-up time for the patients. Usually, no more than six pounds are used during the patient's initial isotonic exercise session to ensure that the patient does not become sore afterwards. Additional isotonic exercises include pulley exercises, weight-well exercises, and exercises with the Bioflex wrist exerciser, the circumferential weightwell, and the work simulator (Figure 20).

Isokinetic exercises performed on exercise equipment such as the Cybex Extremity System 350 improve endurance and general body conditioning. Painless and highly effective, isokinetic exercises are dynamic contractions of muscles with varying degrees of resistance applied by the patient throughout a full range of motion with the speed of movement controlled (Sanders 1984). Isokinetic exercisers can be used to encourage cardiovascular conditioning in addition to upper extremity conditioning. Additional therapeutic equipment includes a Concept II Rowing Ergometer, Nordic Track, Stairmaster 4000, and UBE Ergometer to improve the patient's general body conditioning.

THERAPEUTIC ACTIVITIES

Therapeutic activities that provide beneficial exercises include macrame, ceramics, leatherwork, woodwork, and wood carving. Macrame is used to initiate prehension and reduce edema as the patient works with his or her arms above heart level. Leatherwork is used to improve pinch strength and increase coordination (Figure 21). Ceramics is used to improve the patient's finger flexion, finger extension, or hand strength (Figure 22). Woodworking helps the patient increase hand strength while sustaining a grip on the woodworking sander. Wood carving is the most resistive therapeutic exercise, as it requires repetitive hammering to shape the log into a sculpture. The patients tend to perform the therapeutic activities for longer periods because they become motivated to complete a project. The result is increased

ON-SITE JOB EVALUATION

Patient Name:_____Contact person:_____

Chart #_____Date:_____

Employer:_____Time spent:_____

Address_____Billing done:_____

Phone:_____

Patient diagnosis:_____Dominance_____Inj.ext._____

Job Title:_____

Brief job description:_____

_____

_____

PHYSICAL DEMANDS OF JOB

Lifting: min. weight lifted_____Frequency_____range_____

         max.   _____Frequency_____range_____

         avg.   _____Frequency_____range_____

         Type/size objects lifted:_____

         _____

         Unilateral/bilateral lifting?_____

Carrying: min. weight lifted _____Frequency_____distance____

         max. weight lifted _____   _____   ____

         avg. weight lifted _____   _____   ____

         unilateral/bilateral _____

Reaching: overhead level - yes/no   frequency _____

         shoulder level - yes/no   frequency _____

         waist level   - yes/no   frequency _____

         below waist level -
                        yes/no   frequency _____

         Unilateral/bilateral _____

Pushing/pulling:

         min. weight _____   frequency _____

         max. weight _____   frequency _____

         avg. weight _____   frequency _____

         Cart or hand truck used? Yes/No

Manipulation:

         Gross: objects manipulated: _____

         _____

         Frequency:_____

         Unilateral/bilateral:_____

         Fine: objects manipulated: _____

         _____

         Frequency:_____

         Unilateral/Bilateral:_____

Standing:

Sitting:

Walking:

Climbing:

Reprinted with permission from the Hand Rehabilitation Center, Ltd., Philadelphia, PA.

Figure 18 The therapist utilizes the on-site job evaluation form to document the patient's demands.

Environment: Exposure to chemicals?_____

             Exposure to vibration?_____

             Exposure to extreme temperatures?_____

             Indoor/outdoor:

Tools Used: Frequency   Position
1)_____
2)_____
3)_____
4)_____
5)_____

Comments:_____

_____

_____

Is part-time work available? Yes/No. If yes, describe:_____

_____

Are job mofications allowed? Yes/No. Describe:_____

_____

_____

Other jobs observed?_____

_____

_____

Patient can RTW: regular job - YES/NO
                  full time/part time

Modified Job:_____

Reprinted with permission from the Hand Rehabilitation Center, Ltd., Philadelphia, PA.

Figure 18 *Continued*

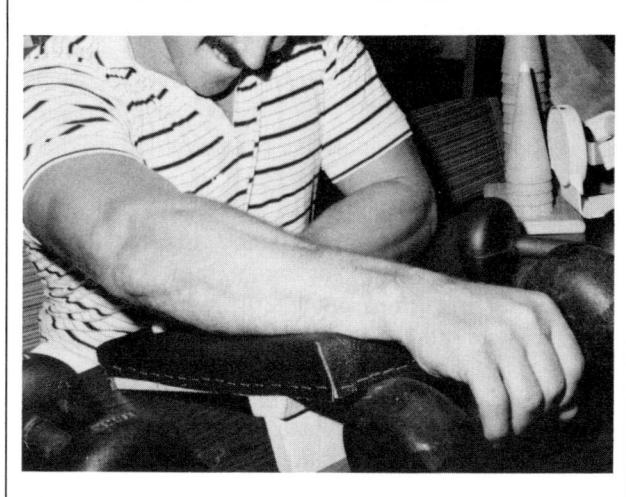

Reprinted with permission from the Hand Rehabilitation Center, Ltd., Philadelphia, PA.

Figure 19 Progressive resistive exercises are performed with three dumbbells to maximize strength rapidly.

endurance through performance (Trombly and Scott 1977).

Job simulation is incorporated in the patient's therapy program as early as possible. The design of a job simulation is based on the information obtained from the occupational interview, job analysis, or on-

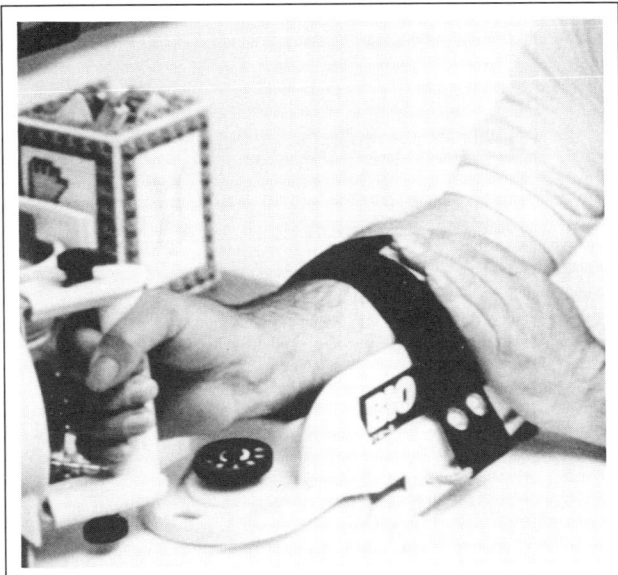

Reprinted with permission from the Hand Rehabilitation Center, Ltd., Philadelphia, PA.

Figure 20 All wrist motions can be performed on the Bio-flex wrist exerciser.

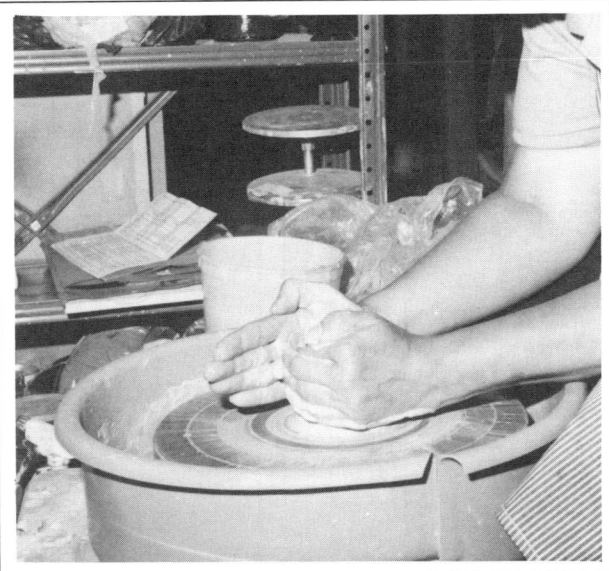

Reprinted with permission from the Hand Rehabilitation Center, Ltd., Philadelphia, PA.

Figure 22 Using a potter's wheel requires controlling the clay by applying resistance with the wrist and finger muscle groups.

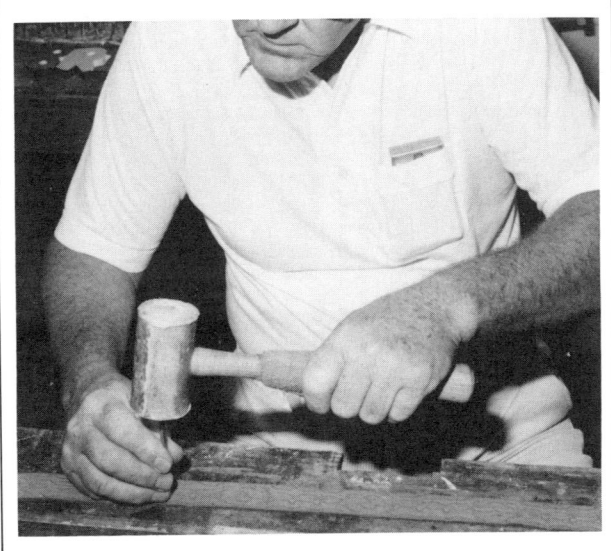

Reprinted with permission from the Hand Rehabilitation Center, Ltd., Philadelphia, PA.

Figure 21 Leatherwork promotes intrinsic muscle strengthening.

site visit. The patient may be required to perform repetitive lifting, carrying, pushing, or pulling. The patient should not lift objects so heavy that swelling or pain results. The weight should be increased gradually as endurance improves. Tool handling is frequently necessary to facilitate the patient's improvement in coordination. The patient may also

focus on increasing general body conditioning through standing while performing therapeutic activities, sitting while exercising, walking, and climbing ladders or stairs as required at work.

RETURN TO WORK PHASE

The Baxter Physical Capacities Evaluation (BPCE) is used to evaluate the patient's physical abilities to perform the requirements of the job. The BPCE includes a hand function evaluation, the administration of standardized tests, and observation of the patient performing the physical demands of the job or the physical demands inherent in any work activity as described in the Smith Physical Capacities Evaluation. Although the evaluation is usually written in a narrative format, a short profile format may be used (Figures 23–25).

Swelling indicates that a patient would have difficulty performing a full eight hours of job tasks successfully. Also, if the patient has difficulty performing any work task, a safe level of performance should be defined and noted by the therapist. If the patient has difficulty lifting, the therapist should note the amount of weight the patient can lift safely without discomfort.

Decreases of sensibility and speed of manipulation should be noted so that the employer can be aware of the patient's need for additional time to complete tasks requiring coordination, such as tool handling.

HAND REHABILITATION CENTER
Philadelphia, PA

PHYSICAL CAPACITIES EVALUATION/SHORT FORM

PATIENT NAME: _____ DATE: _____
PATIENT NUMBER: _____
DIAGNOSIS: _____

Hand Dominance: Right _____ Left _____ Ambidextrous _____
                Changed to R _____ Changed to L _____

Occupation: _____

HAND EVALUATION:

Maximum Grip/Pinch Strength: recorded on Jamar Dynamometer #_____
                             and Pinch Meter

Grip R _____ Level 1 2 3 4 5   Key pinch R _____   Pulp pinch R _____
Grip L _____ Level 1 2 3 4 5   Key pinch L _____   Pulp pinch L _____

Joints Range of Motion/Limitations: _____

Sensibility:

Protective Sensation: R _____ Normal _____ Impaired _____ Absent
Ability to Perceive   L _____ Normal _____ Impaired _____ Absent
Temperature and
Painful Stimuli: R _____ Normal _____ Impaired _____ Absent

Discriminative
Sensation: R _____ Normal _____ Impaired _____ Absent
Ability to Perceive
size, shapes and   L _____ Normal _____ Impaired _____ Absent
textures:

Hand Restrictions: R _____ Normal _____ Left _____ Both _____

Patient can lift/carry: Mark right (R) or left (L) in appropriate box:

Maximum lbs. 5 or 5 10 15 20 25 30 35 40 45 50 55 60 65 70 75 80 above 80 lbs.
             less __ __ __ __ __ __ __ __ __ __ __ __ __ __ __ __ __

Frequently __ __ __ __ __ __ __ __ __ __ __ __ __ __ __ __ __
Occasionally __ __ __ __ __ __ __ __ __ __ __ __ __ __ __ __ __
Never   __ __ __ __ __ __ __ __ __ __ __ __ __ __ __ __ __

Patient can use hands to repetitive: Mark (R) or (L) for each task:
A Simple Grasping   B Pushing & Pulling   C Fine Manipulation

Released to Work: Full Duty Date: _____ Yes _____ No _____   Restricted Duty _____
Comments: _____
Reviewed by therapist _____
Reviewed by surgeon _____

Reprinted with permission from the Hand Rehabilitation Center, Ltd., Philadelphia, PA.

Figure 23 The HRC Physical Capacities Short Profile Form.

HAND REHABILITATION CENTER
Philadelphia, PA

PHYSICAL CAPACITY EVALUATION/LONG FORM

PATIENT NAME: _____ DATE: _____
PATIENT NUMBER: _____
DIAGNOSIS: _____

Hand Dominance: Right _____ Left _____ Ambidextrous _____
                Changed to R _____ Changed to L _____

Occupation: _____

Physical Requirements of Job: _____

I. HAND EVALUATION:

Maximum Grip/Pinch Strength: recorded on Jamar Dynamometer #_____
and Pinch Meter, Grip tested from tight fisted grasp on Level 1 to
wide grasp on Level 5.

Grip R _____ Level 1 2 3 4 5   Key pinch R _____   Pulp pinch R _____
Grip L _____ Level 1 2 3 4 5   Key pinch L _____   Pulp pinch L _____

Joint Range of Motion/Limitations: _____

Sensibility:

Protective Sensation: R _____ Normal _____ Impaired _____ Absent
Ability to perceive
temperature and painful
stimuli.   L _____ Normal _____ Impaired _____ Absent

Discriminative
Sensation: ability-   R _____ Normal _____ Impaired _____ Absent
to perceive size,
shape and textures.   L _____ Normal _____ Impaired _____ Absent

Precautions for Work: _____

Coordination and Dexterity Assessment:

Test Code: T-Tested   C-Contra-indicated   R-Refused

Purdue Pegboard Test   Within   Below
(Measures fingertip dexterity) RUE _____ Normal _____ Normal _____ Unable #_____
                                LUE _____ WN _____ BN _____ Unable #_____

Comments: _____

Reprinted with permission from the Hand Rehabilitation Center, Ltd., Philadelphia, PA.

Figure 24 The HRC Physical Capacities Long Profile Form.

Hand Rehabilitation Center

Phys. Cap. Eval. Long Form

Valpar Whole Body ROM Work Sample Bilateral (Measures ability to perform small manipulative tasks in various body postures)

	Within Normal	Below Normal	Unable	%

Comments: _____

Valpar Simulated Assembly Work Sample (measures reaching, handling and bilateral manipulation of a three part assembly task on a conveyor belt)

	Within Normal	Below Normal	Unable	%

Comments: _____

II. PHYSICAL CAPACITY OBSERVATION:

Test Code: T - Tested   C-Contra-indicated   R - Refused

Patient can reach:

	Within Normal	Below Normal	Unable
RUE			
LUE	WN	BN	Unable

Comments: _____

Patient can lift and carry with right hand:

	Never	Occasionally	Frequently	Continuously
A. 5 lbs or less				
B. Up to 10 lbs.				
C. 11 - 20 lbs.				
D. 21 - 30 lbs.				
E. 31 - 40 lbs.				
F. 41 - 50 lbs.				
G. 51 - 100 lbs.				
H. 100 lbs. and above.				

Comments: _____

Reprinted with permission from the Hand Rehabilitation Center, Ltd., Philadelphia, PA.

Figure 24 *Continued*

Hand Rehabilitation Center

Phys. Cap. Eval. Long Form

Valpar UE ROM Work Sample (measures coordination and manual dexterity of each hand)

	Within Normal	Below Normal	Unable	%
RUE				
LUE				

Comments: _____

Jebsen Hand Function Test (measures coordination as related to activities of daily living)

	Within Normal	Below Normal	Unable	%
RUE				
LUE				

Comments: _____

Valpar Small Tools Mechanical Work Sample (measures coordination and manual dexterity of each hand.)

	Within Normal	Below Normal	Unable	%
RUE				
LUE				

Comments: _____

Handling

Minnesota Rate of Manipulation Test (measures reaching, handling and manipulation)

	Within Normal	Below Normal	Unable	%
RUE				
LUE				

Comments: _____

Reprinted with permission from the Hand Rehabilitation Center, Ltd., Philadelphia, PA.

Figure 24 *Continued*

67

Hand Rehabilitation Center

Phys. Cap. Eval. Long Form

Patient can lift and carry with left hand:

	Never	Occasionally	Frequently	Continuously
A. 5 lbs. or less.				
B. Up to 10 lbs.				
C. 11 - 20 lbs.				
D. 21 - 30 lbs.				
E. 31 - 40 lbs.				
F. 41 - 50 lbs.				
G. 51 - 100 lbs.				
H. 100 lbs. and above.				

Comments:

Patient can push/pull with both hands:

	Never	Occasionally	Frequently	Continuously
A. 5 lbs or less.				
B. Up to 10 lbs.				
C. 11 - 20 lbs.				
D. 21 - 30 lbs.				
E. 31 - 40 lbs.				
F. 41 - 50 lbs.				
G. 51 - 100 lbs.				
H. 100 lbs. and above.				

Comments:

Reprinted with permission from the Hand Rehabilitation Center, Ltd., Philadelphia, PA.

Figure 24 *Continued*

NAME:
CHART:
DATE:
EVALUATOR:

MEDICAL HISTORY AND IDENTIFYING INFORMATION:

This _____ year-old, _____ (right/left) hand dominant (male/female) was employed at _____ (job title) at _____ (co. name). On _____ (date) Mr. _____ (Name) sustained a _____ (crush) -type of injury to the _____ (right/left) both) extremity (ies) resulting in _____ (list of injuries) while at _____ (work or home). Surgery was performed on _____ (date) by Dr. _____ (name). Surgical procedures included: _____ .

Mr. _____ (name) was followed in therapy at _____ (location) for _____ (length of time). At the present time, _____ (name) is _____ (discharged or continues therapy). _____ (name) has not worked since the date of injury. _____ (he/she) attempted to return to work, however, this was unsuccessful.

Mr. _____ (name) indicates that _____ (he/she) is _____ (single, married, divorced, widowed) with _____ (# of children). _____ (He/she) indicates _____ (independence, assistance needed, dependence in self-care and home-care activities). Limitations include: _____

_____

Leisure activities include: _____

Reprinted with permission from the Hand Rehabilitation Center, Ltd., Philadelphia, PA.

Figure 25 The HRC Physical Capacities Evaluation Narrative Form is used with the majority of reports to ensure completeness.

_____ (Mr.Ms.) (name of patient) described the job requirements of _____ (former job) as:

_____ (He/she) indicated the work environment included:

_____ (Name of Patient) reported additional job history included:

Dr. _____ (name) determined that _____ (Mr./Ms.) (name of patient) will be unable to _____ (perform former job or parts of his former job). Dr. _____ (name) ordered the PCE to determine 1. if _____ (Mr./Ms.) (name of patient) can return to his/her present job, 2. to determine Mr./Ms. (name of patient) physical capabilities and limitations and 3. to determine the level of work Mr./Ms. (name of patient) could accomplish given his/her physical abilities and limitations.

The Physical Capacity Evaluation consists of three components: a Hand Function Evaluation, Administration of Standardized Tests, and Observation of Performance of Physical Demands and Job Simulation.

HAND FUNCTION EVALUATION:

Grip strength taken on the Jamar Dynamometer were as follows:

RIGHT HAND _____ lbs.   LEFT HAND _____ lbs.

JAMAR DYNAMOMETER
Level I (tight grip)
Level II
Level III
Level IV
Level V (wide grip)

Figure 25 *Continued*

Mr. _____ (name) has been able/unable to participate in _____ since his injury.

_____ (Mr./Ms. name) indicates _____ (his/her) major difficulties include:

Additional medical history is significant for:

The patient stated he is taking _____ (medication) for _____ (condition).

JOB HISTORY:

Mr./Ms. (name) was employed as a _____ (job title) for _____ (years/months). The Dictionary of Occupational Titles defines this job as _____ (sedentary, light, medium, heavy, very heavy) with the physical demands as:

An On-Site Visit was performed on _____ (date), at _____ (company). _____ Mr./Ms. (name), the _____ (job title) indicated that the job requirements of _____ (job title) included:

At the request of the Hand Rehabilitation Center, _____ (Mr. Ms.) (name), the _____ (job title), completed a job analysis that indicated Mr. _____ (name of patient) job requirements as:

Figure 25 *Continued*

Pinch measurements were recorded with the Pinch Meter. Pinch measurements were as follows:

RIGHT HAND   LEFT HAND

Lateral Pinch:

Palmar pinch

Three-Point Pinch:

Tip Pinch:
thumb/index
thumb/long
thumb/ring
thumb/little

Active Range of Motion measurements were recorded with a goniometer as follows:

Passive range of motion measurements taken with a goniometer are as follows:

Volumetric measurements taken before and after the Physical Capacity Evaluation demonstrated that their _____ (was/was not) a significant increase in hand volume. This indicates that this patient tolerated three hours of manual work without swelling occurring in his hand.

(or) This indicates that this patient did not tolerate the evaluation well, as indicated by increased hand volume.

ADMINISTRATION OF STANDARDIZED TESTS:

The Valpar Upper Extremity Range of Motion Work Sample was utilized to assess the reaching, handling, and manipulating ability of each hand.

Reprinted with permission from the Hand Rehabilitation Center, Ltd., Philadelphia, PA.

Figure 25 *Continued*

This test was performed in a confined space and with vision occluded.

_____ (Name) scored in the _____ (percentile) using the Valpar San Diego Employed Worker Norms for the dominant _____ (right/left) hand.

_____ (He/she) scored in the _____ (percentile) using the Valpar San Diego Employed Worker Norms for the non-dominant _____ (right/left) hand.

This score is a _____ (below average, average, above average) score, as Employed Worker Norms range from 0 to 100%.

COMMENTS:

The Valpar Whole Body Range of Motion Work Sample was used to assess the patient's ability to handle and manipulate objects while working in various body positions including bending, kneeling, and stooping, with vision occluded. _____ (Name) scored in the _____ (#) percentile using the Valpar San Diego Employed Worker Norms. This score is a _____ (below average, average) score as compared to Employed Workers Norms from 0 to 100%.

COMMENTS:

The Valpar Simulated Work Sample assesses the patient's ability to work at an assembly task requiring physical manipulation, as well as bilateral hand usage. _____ (Name) scored in the _____ (#) percentile based upon the Valpar Method Timed Motion Standards. This score is an _____ (below average, average, above average) score in that method timed motion standards range from 0 to 150%.

The Valpar Small Tools Mechanical Work Sample measures a patient's ability to work with small tools.

Reprinted with permission from the Hand Rehabilitation Center, Ltd., Philadelphia, PA.

Figure 25 *Continued*

70

#1) Right Hand -

#2) Left Hand -

#3) Both Hands -

#4) Right plus left plus both hands -

#5) Assembly

COMMENTS:

The Minnesota Rate of Manipulation Test was used to measure the patient's speed of manipulation. On the placing test, the patient scored in the _____ percentile. This is a _____ (below average, average, above average) score since the Minnesota Rate of Manipulation Test is standardized with norms ranging from 0 to 100%. On the turning test, the patient scored in the _____ percentile. This is a _____ score which is compared to the norms ranging from 0 to 100%.

OBSERVATION OF PERFORMANCE OF PHYSICAL DEMANDS OF WORK:

Physical Task:	Observation:
1) Lifting/Carrying	(Name) was able to lift and carry _____ (#) of lbs. with the left arm, _____ (#) of lbs. with the right arm, a distance of 25 ft. _____ (He/she) was able to lift and carry _____ (#) of lbs. with both arms.
2) Pushing/Pulling	(Name) was able to pull _____ (#) of lbs. with the right arm using a wall pulley for _____ (#) of minutes. Using _____ (his/her) left arm (#) of lbs. were pulled for _____ (#) of minutes. (Name) could push and pull a _____ lb. box at waist height repetitively with the right arm for 3 minutes. (He/she) could push and pull a _____ (#) lb. box at waist height repetitively with the left arm for 3 minutes.

Reprinted with permission from the Hand Rehabilitation Center, Ltd., Philadelphia, PA.

Figure 25 *Continued*

---

screwdrivers, nut drivers, Allen wrenches, and various sized wrenches. On the panel requiring _____ tool use, the patient scored in the _____ percentile using San Diego Employed Worker Norms. This score is a _____ (below average, average, above average) score as Employed Worker Norms range from 0 to 100%.

COMMENTS:

The Valpar Drafting Worksample measures a patient's ability to perform clerical skills. _____ (Name) scored in the _____ percentile using Valpar San Diego Employed Worker Norms. This is a _____ (below average, average, above average) score when compared to employed worker norms which range from 0 to 100%. Specific clerical skills were tested and scores for _____ (telephone answering, filing, typing or bookkeeping). Coordination and dexterity were assessed using the Jebson Hand Function Test. This test measures the patient's ability to write, eat, manipulate small lightweight objects, as well as circumferential 1 lb. objects. _____ (Name) scored within normal limits on _____ of the seven (7) test components. _____ (He/she) scored _____ (below normal limits) or (within normal limits) on _____ (writing, simulated eating, stacking, turning, lifting, and placing objects of 1 lb. onto board).

COMMENTS:

The Perdue Pegboard Test was utilized to measure fingertip dexterity. Five separate scores are obtained from the Perdue Pegboard as follows:

Reprinted with permission from the Hand Rehabilitation Center, Ltd., Philadelphia, PA.

Figure 25 *Continued*

3) Reaching

____ (Name) was able to reach forward (with no difficulty/with some difficulty). ____ (He/she) was able to reach overhead ____ (with difficulty/without difficulty). ____ (He/she) was able to reach down (with or without difficulty).

Endurance was ____ (Poor, fair, good) for reaching. ____ (Name) was able to extend arms in a reaching task for ____ minutes (with difficulty/without difficulty).

4) Grasping/Handling

____ (Name) can use right hand for grasping and handling of ____ (small, light, heavy-sized objects) without difficulty/with difficulty. ____ (He/she) can utilize the left hand for grasping and handling of ____ (small, light, heavy) sized objects (with/without difficulty).

5) Manipulation

Fine manipulation was ____ (within normal limits or below normal limits) with the right hand. Left hand manipulation was ____ (within normal limits or below normal limits).

6) Standing, Sitting, Walking

Standing tolerance is estimated to be ____ hours. Walking tolerance is estimated to be ____ miles. Sitting tolerance is estimated to be ____ hours. There was ____ abnormal, normal, date and body posture observed.

7) Climbing Stairs/Ladders

____ (Name) was able to climb stairs, (with without difficulty.) He/she was able to climb a ladder ____ (with/without difficulty)

8) Kneeling, Crouching, Crawling, Stooping

____ (Name) was able to kneel, crouch, stoop and crawl ____ (frequently, occasionally, infrequently).

9) Endurance

Endurance was tested using the work Simulator. It is a computerized evaluation instrument that can measure the amount of power emitted by the hands and arms with a variety of tools. The test compares tool use between hands for a three-minute period. With the tool that simulates (motion, tool or job demand) ____ (his/her) right or left hand showed ____ # percentile less of or more power than his ____ hand.

With the next tool that simulates ____ (tool, motion, or jor requirement) ____ his/her left or right showed ____ # percentile less or more power as compared to his ____ (right or left). With the tool that simulates ____ (job, tool, motion) endurance measured ____ (#) percentile ____ (greater or lesser) in the ____ (right or left) arm than the (right or left) arm.

RECOMMENDATIONS:

Based on the ____ (Name) test response, it is recommended that he/she) can perform work ____ (Part-time or full-time) with the following restrictions:

P/T	F/T	
____	____	Sedentary work - including 10 lbs. maximum lifting and/or carrying articles walking/standing intermittently.
____	____	Light work including 25 lbs. maximum lifting carrying 10 lb. articles frequently. Most jobs involve sitting with a degree of pushing and pulling.
____	____	Medium work - 50 lbs. maximum lifting with frequent lifting/carrying of up to 25 lbs. Frequent standing and walking.
____	____	Heavy work - 75 lbs. maximum lifting with frequent lifting/carrying of up to 50 lbs.
____	____	Frequent standing and walking -
____	____	Very heavy work, lifting objects over 100 lbs. and frequent lifting/carrying of 75 lbs. or more.

COMMENTS: _____

_____

_____

_____

Therapist's signature _____

Physician's signature _____ Date: _____

Reprinted with permission from the Hand Rehabilitation Center, Ltd., Philadelphia, PA.

Figure 25 *Continued*

72

Reprinted with permission from the Hand Rehabilitation Center, Ltd., Philadelphia, PA.

Figure 25 *Continued*

If the job requires rapid manipulation, the patient may be unable to perform specific manipulation tasks.

Communication with the employer is an ongoing process. Discussion with the employer or personnel manager in regard to the job analysis or during the on-site visit creates a cooperative relationship for negotiations when the patient is ready to return to work. Initially, the personnel manager may feel that no other work is possible if the patient cannot return to the regular job. However, the therapist may negotiate for the patient to return to work part of the day on the regular job and part of the day on a modified job.

The employer may allow the patient to work part time initially, to ensure that the patient can perform the job adequately as his or her endurance increases. It is important to educate the personnel manager about the patient's abilities as well as restrictions. The personnel manager must be reminded of the patient's assets in order to facilitate the patient's return to work.

If the patient cannot perform the regular job, and the employer does not have modified work available, the patient may need to change jobs. The patient is referred to a vocational placement service or vocational evaluation service. The therapist can help by contacting the insurance company and explaining the need for vocational placement.

The completed evaluation of the patient's physical capacities is sent to the vocational placement office to outline the patient's physical abilities and restrictions. The therapist should state the level of work the patient can attain, based on the definitions in the *DOT*. The therapist should state whether the patient can perform sedentary work (up to 10 lb. of lifting), light work (up to 25 lb. of lifting), medium work (up to 50 lb. of lifting), heavy work (up to 100 lb. of lifting), or very heavy work (lifting in excess of 100 lb.).

The vocational placement office is encouraged to communicate with the therapist when job possibilities arise. The therapist may discuss with the vocational placement counselor the possibility of the patient's successfully performing modified alternative jobs. The therapist can correlate the physical demands of the modified jobs with the patient's physical abilities and recommend the patient for specific jobs. However, it is the duty of the rehabilitation specialist or vocational placement counselor to suggest specific jobs that are available in the community. Only these individuals have the requisite knowledge of the available labor market.

REFERENCES

Ballard, M., Baxter, P., Bruening, L. and Fried, S. "Work Therapy and Return to Work." In Mackin, E. (Ed.) *Hand Clinics*, Vol. 2, No. 1, Philadelphia: W. B. Saunders, 1986.

Gimby, G., Heinje, C., Von Hook, O. and Wedel, H. "Muscle Strength and Endurance after Training with Repeated Maximal Isometric Contraction." *Scandinavian Journal Rehabilitation Medicine* 5 (1973) 118–23.

Sanders, M.T. "A Comparison of Two Methods of Training on the Development of Muscular Strength and Endurance," *Journal of Orthopedic and Sports Physical Therapy* (December 1984): 210–13.

Trombly, C. and Scott, A. *Occupational Therapy for Physical Dysfunction*, Baltimore: Williams and Wilkins, 1977.

U.S. Dept. of Labor. *Dictionary of Occupational Titles*, 5th ed. Washington, DC: U.S. Government Printing Office, 1991.

Zinovieff, A.N. "Heavy-Resistance Exercises, The Oxford Technique," *The British Journal* (June 1951) 129–32.

CHAPTER FIVE

USE OF THE PHYSICAL CAPACITIES EVALUATION IN THE INDUSTRIAL MODEL

THERAPISTS WORKING AS INDUSTRIAL CONSULtants offer services for primary or secondary prevention of industrial injuries or cumulative trauma disorders. Primary prevention efforts are aimed at preventing injury-producing events (Ellexson 1985–86). Secondary prevention activities focus on early detection of dysfunction and the provision of appropriate intervention to prevent progression to a more chronic condition (West 1969).

The education of occupational therapists in human anatomy, kinesiology, physiology, neurology, and pathology equips them with the knowledge to analyze the physical components of jobs and the methods of job performance that can lead to neuromuscular and musculoskeletal problems. The therapist attempts to fit the work to the worker by analyzing the situation and making cost-effective, realistic suggestions to employees and management. The employees benefit because they are assisted in their efforts to work more efficiently with less risk of injury. The employer benefits because the incidence of occupational injuries and disorders is reduced, thereby reducing costs for medical care and time lost from work.

Therapists working in the industrial model of practice are pioneers. The work is satisfying when their services facilitate the healthy population to continue working at their optimal level. At other times, a perplexing adversarial attitude on the part of both employees and employers may thwart the therapists from providing anything more than suggestions. However, therapists who like to travel, meet people, work independently, and provide nontraditional therapeutic intervention may find industrial consultation quite rewarding.

REFERRAL SOURCES

Referrals are obtained by several methods. Therapists who provide industrial consultation should learn how to market themselves and make professional sales presentations, because these considerations often determine whether they will be hired. The job of selling oneself may be uncomfortable; however, it is absolutely necessary. For starters, a professional-looking resume and business cards are essential. In addition, the therapist needs to know the nature of each business in order to describe the services that can be provided to benefit the company.

It is crucial to sell to upper management, as upper management has the authority to secure cooperation from middle management. The therapist should present several proposals ranging from a one-time ergonomic analysis of work stations to weekly evaluations of the postural alignment of workers at the stations. The financial benefit of investing in the prevention of injury should be emphasized by citing examples in the literature (Ellexson 1985–86, Lepore et al. 1984, Morris 1984). The advantages of developing consultation services with upper management are numerous. Among the most important is that the therapist may be able to work with personnel from the manufacturing, safety, and engineering departments to make whatever changes are necessary successfully. The cooperation of each department will be mandated by upper management.

Occasionally, ergonomic engineers from the engineering department will request specific information on medical disorders that might result from improperly designed machines or ergonomically stressful methods of job performance. The ergonomic engineer knows the details about machine design to effect appropriate modification. But the therapist can analyze what movements aggravate musculoskeletal structures and suggest further modifications. Together, the therapist and ergonomic engineer can implement minor changes in the design of the work station that can make the worker more productive.

Many times, referrals are obtained after the therapist has spoken at a professional meeting for occupational health nurses, occupational medicine physicians, insurance companies, or rehabilitation companies. When referrals come from medical department staff at the industrial site, the medical director or occupational health nurse director may request educational lectures to the medical staff and the employees on the prevention of injuries and management of cumulative trauma disorders. The director may request consultation to place injured workers in appropriate modified jobs. Also, the therapist may be asked to develop an exercise program for the employees.

INDICATIONS OF THE NEED FOR SERVICES

A physical capacities evaluation is used in primary intervention for reintegrating the injured worker into the workplace. Such an evaluation is also used to educate workers and management about work practices that could result in injuries.

When a worker is injured, rehabilitation may be lengthy. Other workers and managers may not understand the worker's lengthy absence or residual physical limitations. Before the injured worker returns to work, a physical capacities evaluation should be completed, with the information shared with management so that it understands how to work with the injured worker.

If the injured worker cannot perform the job safely for a full shift, the employer should be told. It is beneficial to speak to the personnel manager or plant manager who determines what job the worker will perform on a daily basis. Management must be educated regarding the patient's physical restrictions.

To ensure adequate communication, it is productive to meet with plant management. Frequently, the injured worker and a union representative attend the meeting, as well as the personnel manager, plant manager, and foreman. Occasionally, a rehabilitation specialist will attend also.

The therapist is concerned with returning the patient to a job that will not result in further injury. To meet this concern the patient must be capable of performing all the physical tasks of the job. If the patient is unable to perform one part of the job—for example, heavy lifting—the therapist asks whether

assistance can be provided for that task. If assistance is unavailable, then other available jobs in the plant are reviewed.

Most companies do not offer light duty. Thus, physicians should not discharge injured workers to return to light duty. Instead, the therapist should ask the plant manager or personnel manager to describe the regular jobs that are available at the plant and then compare the job requirements to the injured worker's abilities. The therapist should recommend placement in a regular job within the range of the injured worker's capacities.

Job rotations are sometimes the solution for placement of the injured worker. The patient may not have adequate endurance to perform the regular job for a full shift. The plant manager may then allow the injured worker to work on the regular job part of the shift and rotate to a less demanding job for the rest of the shift. The therapist can make these recommendations after completing a physical capacities evaluation and an on-site visit.

The therapist checks with the personnel manager once a month to determine the injured worker's success on the job. The employer may request a repeat of the physical capacities evaluation to see whether the patient has gained endurance or strength.

A therapist may administer a physical capacities evaluation to an injured worker as many as four times over a period of three years. With each evaluation, if the performance of the injured worker improves, he or she may be able to be transferred to a job that is more demanding (see Industrial Reports, Chapter 8).

Lectures on safety are considered part of the therapist's primary intervention. Employees who see slide presentations demonstrating the kinds of injuries machines can cause tend to practice safe work habits. It is important to educate assembly line workers, computer operators, and other workers on the motions and postures that can lead to inflammation of tendons and nerves and result in cumulative trauma disorders. Workers should be taught to avoid the repetitive stress caused by these working postures.

Therapists may lecture once in a facility, but continued communication with managers may lead to secondary efforts. Primary and secondary prevention efforts at each industrial site are most beneficial. Figure 1 contains a report on industrial consultation that provides continued communications.

THE PHYSICAL CAPACITIES EVALUATION IN SECONDARY INTERVENTION

The physical capacities evaluation measures the worker's tolerance by measuring hand volume, strength, coordination, and endurance. If swelling occurs or the worker fails to complete the physical capacities evaluation, then the therapist initiates secondary prevention activities.

The therapist teaches the patient to use less stressful postures while working. For example, a computer operator typing with wrists flexed can develop carpal tunnel syndrome, and an assembler in an automotive plant repetitively pounding metal panels into place with the palm can cause ulnar nerve compression at Guyon's canal.

Teaching workers to change posture is most ef-

COMPANY

April 17, 1986

TO: E.F.   P 56–35

CC: B.F.   P 31–03
                  P.   Jefferson Hand Center
                  L.   P 50–19
                  G.M.   P 30–46
C.M.   P 50–02

Subject: Prevention of Hand Injuries in Wire Shop

On April 15, 1986, Jefferson University Hand Center gave a presentation to the Company Medical Department personnel on the anatomy, physiology, and symptomatology of carpal tunnel syndrome. Also included was the prevention and treatment of the carpal tunnel syndrome. A presentation by Hand Clinic personnel on hand tools and their proper use, proper body mechanics, ergonomics of the job, and exercising of the neck and hands while at the job site was given to the first- and second-shift female employees of the Wire Shop. There was also a question and answer period. There were 45 female employees present from 2:15 p.m. to 3:03 p.m. for the first presentation and 25 female employees present from 3:45 p.m. to 4:28 p.m. for the second presentation. There was a total of 54.75 hours of this presentation.

I am sending you 104 hand safety booklets, tendon gliding exercise papers, and neck and hand exercise papers for your first-line supervisors and the remainder of your employees who did not attend the presentations.

Employees who attended the meeting responded that they were very receptive and that the presentation would be helpful. Some enthusiastically participated in the exercise portion of the program. Some employees complained at the time that the tools they were using were from 1966 and were hurting their hands, and that some of the tools sent for calibration were returned the same way they were sent. In my conversation with you today, April 17, the "complaints" were discussed. There are some tools in the shop that are from 1966; however, they do meet the criteria for the job. If the tool is hurting the hand, then another tool should be obtained by the employee, or the tool could be padded. When a tool is sent for a calibration tool test, the tool must meet such requirements as "go, no go gage, the crib terminals and lugs, and the pool test" to pass the said test. Sometimes a tool does meet all the requirements and returns to the shop without any adjustments.

Sometimes a tool is adjusted and returned, and sometimes a tool is scrapped and a replacement is bought. Maybe if the employee understood this calibration process, the concerns would disappear.

We have purchased the slide presentation from the Jefferson Hand Center, and whenever the need arises, we will present the same program to the employees throughout the shop.

I am recommending to you that first-line supervisors encourage employees to do hand and neck exercises. Thank you for your cooperation. I hope this will reduce the hand injury problems in your shop.

If there are any questions, please call me at x 3370.

Manager, Health Services

HVH/mb
2–THUR

Figure 1.

fective if the instruction is repeated frequently. The therapist arranges to consult once a week or twice a month at each plant. At the plant, the therapist walks around, talks to workers, and gains their confidence. If a worker is seen using a stressful posture, the therapist consults with the worker immediately (James 1985). This type of intervention prevents many workers from developing chronic conditions.

An occupational therapist can suggest a modification to either the work site or work methods by using the job analysis section of the physical capacities evaluation to identify those parts of the job that cause physiological stress. For example, one company requested a consultation due to the high incidence of thoracic outlet syndrome in its bacon-wrapping department. In a job analysis and on-site visit, the therapist noticed that the height of the upper conveyor belt required most of the female packers to reach to approximately 120 degrees of shoulder flexion and bend their wrists 30 degrees to grasp the pound of bacon they were packing. Based on a knowledge of causes of thoracic outlet syndrome and carpal tunnel syndrome, the therapist recommended lowering the upper conveyor belt by six inches. Following this modification, the number of complaints diminished significantly.

A simple modification to the work site is a change in chair height so as to permit workers' feet to rest flat on the floor or on a foot support (Figure 2.A). Other modifications may be just as simple. Work surfaces can be tilted so that workers looking into microscopes do not have to flex their necks forward. Pneumatic tools can be installed to replace hand tools. Well-fitting gloves can be worn to decrease friction applied to the flexor tendons. Armrests, wristrests, and back supports decrease stress on the seated computer operator.

A thorough review of the literature on ergonomics prepares the way for the therapist to intervene in regard to modifying the methods of performing work. Certain motions have been cited as stressful to the upper extremity (Armstrong et al. 1982, Tichauer and Gage 1977, Tichauer 1978). For example, pinching and flexing the wrist increases pressure in the carpal tunnel (Kirkbeck and Beer 1975), and carpal tunnel syndrome can result if these motions are repeated. Ulnar deviation of the wrist can result in De Quervain's syndrome (Luopajarvi et al. 1979) (Figure 2.B).

The therapist breaks down each job by analyzing the physical movements required for the performance of the job. If stressful movements are involved, the therapist suggests changes in accordance with the rules of ergonomics. For example, it is better for workers to keep their wrists straight or slightly

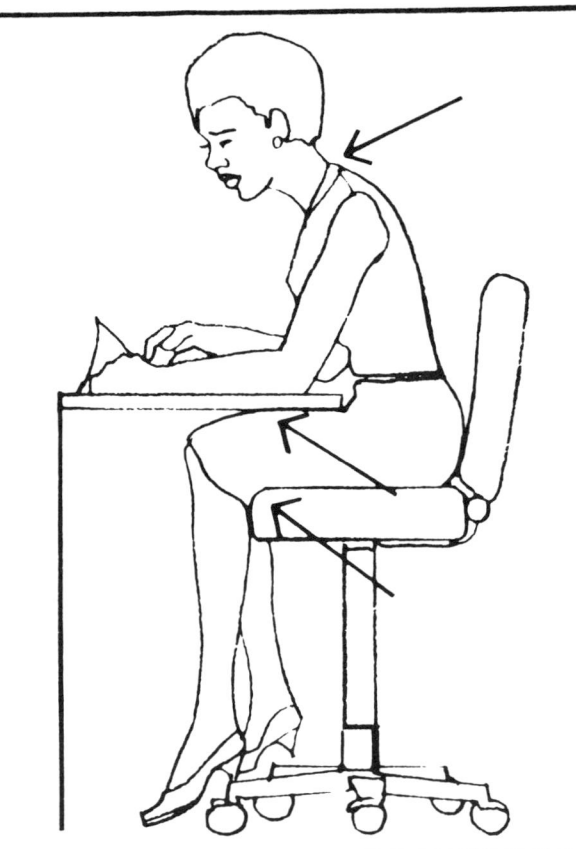

Figure 2.A   This employee's stressful postures included forwardly flexed neck, unsupported back, and unsupported feet. (Courtesy of The Travelers Insurance Companies.)

dorsiflexed while working. It also is better to use tools with long curved handles rather than tools with short handles that cause compression of tendons and nerves in the palm (Figure 3).

If a work task requires wrist flexion as the worker reaches forward for objects, the work task should be positioned to the side of the worker to allow him or her to perform the task with the forearm and wrist in neutral.

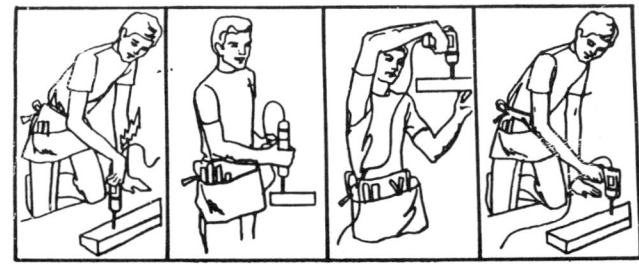

Figure 2.B.   Minor changes in the work station, work method, or tools can alleviate musculoskeletal strain in workers. (Courtesy of The Travelers Insurance Companies.)

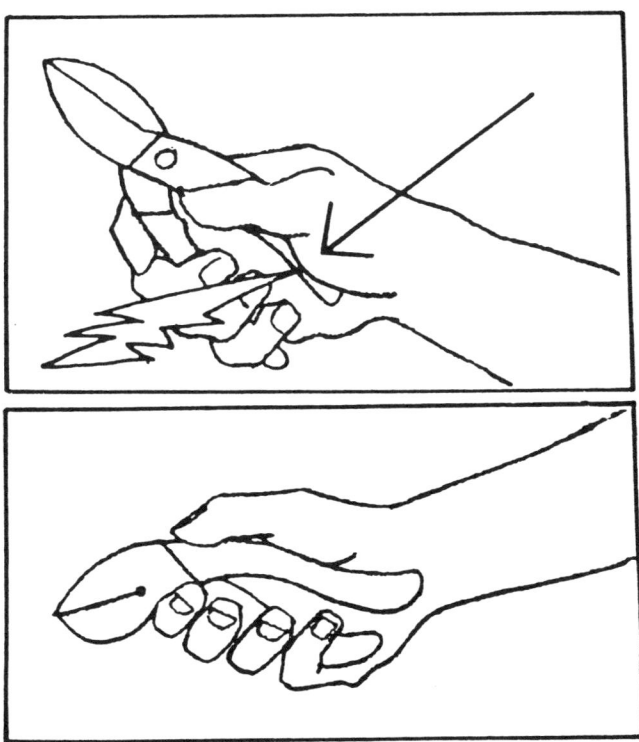

Figure 3. It is better to use tools with long curved handles. (Courtesy of The Travelers Insurance Companies.)

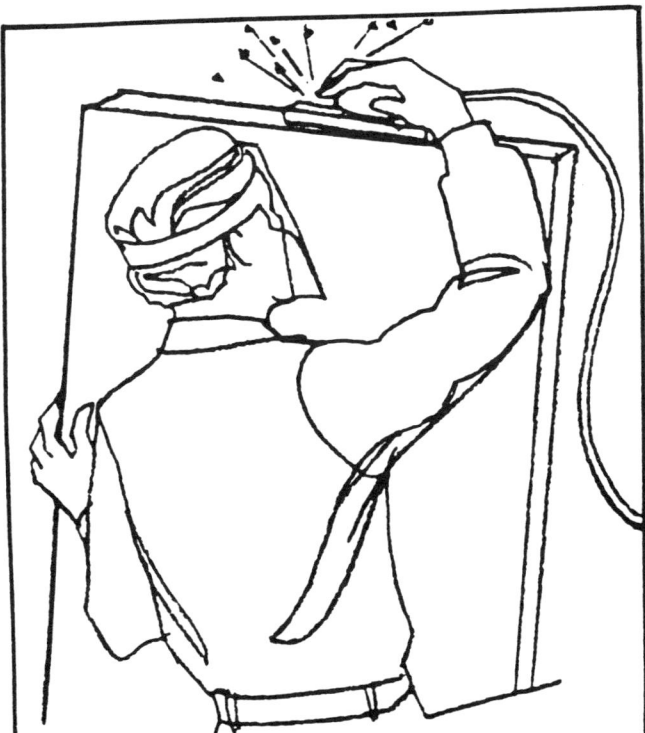

Figure 5. This employee could decrease reaching by standing on a platform. (Courtesy of The Travelers Insurance Companies.)

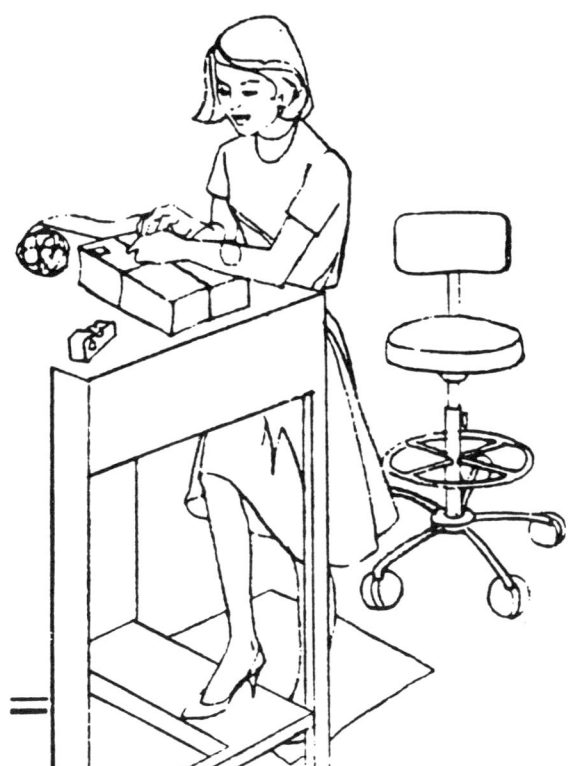

Figure 4. Armrests and footrests decrease fatigue and enable the worker to work comfortably. (Courtesy of The Travelers Insurance Companies.)

Simple modifications are often all that is necessary. The thousands of dollars spent to retrofit a machine may not be as cost effective as building armrests, footrests, or supports to position the worker for a few hundred dollars (Figure 4). The least expensive modification is teaching workers to limit repetitive wrist flexion and ulnar deviation or to avoid shoulder stress by limiting prolonged reaching with the arms unsupported. Employees may decrease reaching by standing on a platform (Figure 5).

It is hard for both workers and management to accept modifications, so the therapist should continue to consult with each organization periodically for at least six months. Such a schedule, though not always possible, is preferred. It is very gratifying to treat a worker's condition with a conservative method and prevent the condition from becoming chronic.

Secondary intervention can be supplied in a clinical setting if the therapist cannot travel to the plant. Workers can be referred by the occupational health nurse or the plant physician. Evaluation and education of the worker can be done before or after work hours. The therapist teaches the worker how to control inflammation and perform stretching and strengthening exercises, and to avoid motions that are irritating (see Industrial Reports, Chapter 8). However, if conservative management does not eliminate inflammation, the worker may need to stop working temporarily and undergo further medical intervention.

Surgery for carpal tunnel syndrome, tennis elbow, and trigger finger can alleviate painful symptoms. However, the therapist should teach the patient to change work postures, take breaks when offered, and control inflammation should the conditions recur. These practices work toward preventing a recurrence of cumulative trauma.

REFERENCES

Armstrong, T. J., Foulke, J. A., Joseph, B. S., and Goldstein, S. A. "Investigation of Cumulative Trauma Disorders in a Poultry Processing Plant." *American Industrial Hygiene Association Journal*, 43 (1982):103–16.

Ellexson, M. "The Unique Role of the Occupational Therapist in Industry." *Occupational Therapy in Health Care*, 2 (1985–86):35–46.

James, S. "Bodies Talk in Ergonomics." *Greensboro News and Record*, Monday, April 8, 1985.

Kirkbeck, M. Q., and Beer, T. C. "Occupation in Relation to the Carpal Tunnel Syndrome." *Rheumatology and Rehabilitation*, 14 (1975):218–21.

Lepore, B. A., Olson, C. N., and Tomer, G. N. "The Dollars and Sense of Occupational Bank Insurance Prevention Training." *Clinical Management in Physical Therapy*, 4 (1984):38–42.

Luopajarvi, T., Kuorinka, I., Virolainen, M., and Holmberg, M. "Prevalence of Tenosynovitis and Other Injuries of the Upper Extremities in Repetitive Work." *Scandinavian Journal of Work, Environment, and Health*, Supplement 3 (1979) 48–55.

Morris, A. "Program Compliance Key to Preventing Low Back Injuries." *Occupational Health and Safety* (March 1984) 44–47.

Tichauer, E. R. *The Biomechanical Basis of Ergonomics: Anatomy Applied to the Design of Work Stations*, New York: John Wiley and Sons, 1978.

Tichauer, E. R. and Gage. "Ergonomic Principles Basic to Hand Tool Design." *American Industrial Hygiene Association Journal*, 28 (November 1977): 622–34.

West, W. A. "The Growing Importance of Prevention." *American Journal of Occupational Therapy*, 23 (1969):226–31.

CHAPTER SIX

THE SMITH PHYSICAL CAPACITIES EVALUATION IN THE LEGAL MODEL

IN RECENT YEARS IN THE LEGAL PROFESSION, IN both trial practice and settlement negotiations, creative approaches have expanded the panel of experts that attorneys select for opinions in personal injury matters (Smith 1984). Attorneys often seek occupational therapists for expertise in assessing functional capacities.

With the many complexities of life today, there is an increasing need for individuals to use legal services. Today, people have to pay for not only the material things, but also for the many natural resources that were easily accessible in the past. Those who do not work must have a source of income. A number of earned benefits in compensation are available to disabled workers, but obtaining those benefits may require legal assistance.

In the socio-legal model of practice, the therapist's services are confined to assisting in substantiating or disqualifying claims for monetary benefits and establishing amicable settlements of insurance claims or damages and lawsuits. Referrals are made for evaluation to establish an individual's level of functional ability and make recommendations for further medical or therapeutic services. These services are extended if the therapist's testimony will be required in the future.

A functional evaluation is routinely administered with the Smith Physical Capacities Evaluation, either alone or in conjunction with other measures of performance. Upon the recommendation of the therapist, the individual who has been evaluated may be referred to a physician for treatment. However, strictly speaking, services in the legal model are confined to functional evaluation (Osterweis et al. 1987) to determine the client's physical abilities and restrictions.

REFERRAL SOURCES

Attorney

Customarily, occupational therapists have collaborated with physicians to provide both evaluation services and treatment of referrals made by physicians. In the legal model of practice, there is a parallel relationship between the therapist and the attorney. Referrals made by attorneys are chiefly for evaluation and consultation in regard to an individual's physical, cognitive, and emotional capabilities to engage in both work activities and activities of daily living. As this area of practice has existed only for about the last 20 years, there is a need to educate the attorney about the occupational therapist's background and area of expertise. Unlike the physician, the attorney most often is unaware of the therapist's medical and behavioral background. Rather, attorneys are generally more impressed with the ocupational therapist's expertise in evaluating a person's functional capacities and communicating these findings in lay terms applicable to the level of activity in the individual's own lifestyle. The word *occupation* further conveys a meaning of vocation, which the attorney equates with work.

In the legal model of practice, the therapist is most often considered a vocational expert, along with others in the specialty disciplines of vocational counseling, vocational evaluation, vocational placement, ergonomic engineering, physiatrics, industrial psychology, and employment counseling. As a result, the therapist must aid the attorney in distinguishing among the expertise of the occupational therapist and that of the other special disciplines, in order that the attorney best use the services of the therapist.

The referring attorney may be representing an

allegedly harmed client or a claimant of benefits. Conversely, the attorney may be representing the adversarial side or defending party. Broadly speaking, the attorney who represents the individual's interest is the plaintiff attorney, and the opposing attorney is the defense attorney.

In general, more plaintiff attorneys than defense attorneys make referrals to occupational therapists. This one-sidedness appears to be due to the desire on the part of many defense attorneys to represent insurance companies in personal injury litigation. More often than not, the therapist finds that his or her counterpart is a rehabilitation specialist or insurance claims investigator. The reason for this seems to be that many insurance companies have a vested interest in subsidiary private vocational rehabilitation companies (Anderson 1979), which rarely employ occupational therapists. The services of these companies are limited mostly to vocational evaluation and vocational rehabilitation case management.

Judges and Administrative Law Judges

In some cases, a judge will specify that attorneys must have a vocational expert's opinion if, in the judge's mind, the question of an individual's return to work has not been adequately addressed. In these instances, an expert who is known to both sides and who is known to give an objective opinion will be called for evaluation and an opinion. In this manner, both parties to the dispute will have the information that is necessary to arrive at an equitable settlement.

Insurance Adjusters and Rehabilitation Nurses

The second largest number of referrals in the legal model of practice come from insurance adjusters and rehabilitation nurses who are involved in claims by insured persons who have suffered personal injury. Except for long-term or difficult claims, these individuals are generally seen more in the rehabilitation model of practice. However, when medical and rehabilitation efforts begin to be exhausted, and the claim has not been resolved, a final legal opinion is sometimes required. A final legal opinion spurs on the insured to take steps to resolve the claim when he or she is seen to have reached the maximum medical benefit and rehabilitation potential.

As before, the scope of services desired by insurance adjusters and rehabilitation nurses is limited. The physical capacities evaluation of the individual's ability to engage in work and daily life activity is one service requested. If recommendations have been made for further rehabilitation, then therapy services are often requested to ready the individual for work.

Self

Although most people seek the counsel of an attorney in matters of substantiating claims for benefits, it often is not necessary to be represented by an attorney in such proceedings. Some individuals choose to self-educate themselves as to the criteria they will have to meet in order to prosecute their claims successfully. They will then go about developing their file and documenting the matters to be addressed. In these cases, the individual often will request a physical capacities or functional capacities evaluation. Frequently, such cases involve appeal claims for social security disability benefits or documentation of disability for insurance claim benefits under a disability insurance policy.

INDICATIONS OF THE NEED FOR SERVICES

Forensic

Common types of litigation for which attorneys seek the services of a therapist involve resulting personal injury or residual medical impairment. Among the causes of such legal action are (1) personal injury (occurring at home, at work, in a vehicle, etc.), (2) alimony payments, (3) product liability damages, (4) social security disability claim appeals, (5) breaches of contract (e.g.,disability insurance contracts), and (6) worker's compensation benefit appeals. In the adversarial system, the cause of action which the plaintiff (the allegedly harmed party) brings must be decided. If the defendant is at fault, he or she must compensate the plaintiff monetarily, to the degree of harm incurred.

Therapists can present testimony pertaining to the damage aspect of a case. Such testimony assists the jury in making an amicable award if liability is found. Most often, consolidated cases are heard, i.e., cases in which issues of liability and damages are heard together. The jury must decide liability first and then the amount of damages.

Each attorney attempts to diminish and discredit the testimony of the opposing attorney. The therapist's objective findings from a physical capacities evaluation, and the opinion based upon these findings, is helpful to both sides, because both the individual's abilities and limitations abilities are described.

Litigation due to a controversy is the action of last resort. Even if a suit is filed, attempts at settlement will continue until the matter is resolved. Negotiations usually continue up until the time of the trial, and sometimes even while the trial progresses. The written report of the occupational therapist is often helpful in bringing the negotiations to a conclusion.

Administrative Proceedings

Administrative hearings and insurance settlement negotiations frequently benefit from opinions based upon functional and physical capacities evaluations. Administrative hearings determine whether a claimant meets the criteria for receiving certain monetary benefits, such as social security disability payments, workers' compensation, civil service disability retirement payments, and longshoreman and harbor workers' benefits.

Since the detailed criteria of a particular law or regulation must be addressed, the therapist should be aware of these criteria. The attorney is often helpful in explaining them and therapists should have copies of the regulations or laws for their reference.

DOCUMENTATION AND REPORTING FORMATS

Unlike the rehabilitation model, reporting in lay language rather than medical terminology is essential in the legal model. Documentation of the findings of the evaluation, opinions drawn, and recommendations based on the findings must be presented in one or more of the following ways:

Sworn testimony is presented before a law judge or an administrative law judge and can be presented in court, in an administrative hearing room, or by means of a videotape deposition (extramural), for purposes of perpetuation or for purposes of discovery.

Oral reports are presented in a hearing room before a hearing officer, committee, or panel.

Written reports include actual litigation, insurance settlements, and reports on hearings on administrative proceedings.

Any one type, or a combination of types, of reporting may be requested. Except in rare instances when specifically requested not to, the therapist issues a written report to the referring party. At a later date, testimony or oral presentation may be requested or subpoenaed.

When testimony is given, the therapist is called as an expert witness. Unlike the eyewitness, the expert witness is able not only to report what he or she observed, but also to give informed opinions based on findings. Preliminary to giving testimony, the therapist must be accepted by the court as an expert witness.

In the process of qualifying as an expert witness, the therapist is requested to explain his or her area of expertise (occupational or physical therapy) and present professional credentials. The opposing attorney then has an opportunity to ask the therapist questions related to credentials and qualifications, and the judge may also ask questions. The opposing attorney may object that the therapist lacks the necessary qualifications in the tendered discipline (or a specific area, for example, occupational or physical therapy). The judge will then either sustain the objection or accept the therapist as an expert.

In giving testimony, the therapist should attempt to speak directly to the jury or judge as directed. The therapist should have reviewed the client's record prior to giving testimony, even though, except in a few instances, he or she will be allowed to refer to notes and reports. At times, the therapist will be requested to read directly from a report or notes. The importance of having a complete and objective report and comprehensive notes is readily understood in view of the fact that the therapist may have to testify months, or even a few years, after seeing the patient.

It is of the utmost importance for the therapist to present testimony in a sincere, credible manner. Following are some guidelines to convey this image:

1. Be well prepared, as a result of having reviewed the patient's record and discussed the testimony with the attorney before the trial.
2. Be relaxed and confident. Do not take any questioning personally. Remember, the judicial system is an adversarial system, with opposing sides attempting to emphasize or deemphasize the testimony.
3. Never be persuaded to change any opinion that is based on your objective findings.
4. Feel free to explain your answers in a concise and meaningful way. Do not ramble, and use lay terms.
5. Never bluff or guess in attempting to answer the question. State honestly that you do not know the answer or that the information is not available.
6. Dress in a professional manner.

A subpoena may be issued to order a therapist to testify at a trial. The subpoena will state the date and time to appear in court. Generally, as a courtesy, the lawyer who has issued the subpoena will not expect the therapist to appear for the duration of the trial. Rather, the lawyer will let the therapist know when to arrive. This arrangement makes it less disruptive for the therapist's schedule.

In the event that the therapist will be unavailable for a trial, a deposition can be taken to substitute for the therapist in the court proceedings in order to present and perpetuate the testimony. The deposition may be reported by videotape or a stenographic transcript. Depositions are generally taken at the therapist's office or some other agreed upon location. The witness is sworn to tell the truth by the videotape reporter or the stenographic reporter. All objections to any part of the deposition raised by attorneys are ruled upon by the judge at the time of the trial. Whenever objections are sustained by the judge, that part of the testimony will be deleted from the court proceedings. Some therapists find depositions less stressful then presenting testimony in court, because of the informality of the office environment. Other therapists prefer to testify in court, since the judge is present to rule at the time of any objection. In-court testimony avoids the possibility of any attorney going beyond the reasonable bounds of questioning.

Depositions taken in court are used for perpetuation of a witness's testimony. At other times, a deposition may be requested of the therapist for the purpose of discovery. This is done when an opposing attorney wishes either to learn what the therapist's findings have been, to educate himself about the area of expertise of the witness, or to see the demeanor of the witness. The deposition is conducted in the same manner as that for perpetuation, except that a stenographic record will be the only document involved, and the scope of questioning may be much broader than in the deposition for perpetuation.

Testimony given for proceedings before an administrative law judge may be in a courtroom or a hearing room. A hearing room atmosphere is less formal than that of a courtroom. The witness is examined and cross-examined by the attorneys, and the judge frequently asks questions of the witness.

In an oral report, the proceedings are much less formal than court proceedings. Nevertheless, the therapist must be prepared and confident. The therapist reports his or her findings to the hearing committee, whose members may then ask questions of the therapists. Oral reports are not adversary proceedings; rather, they are intended to determine whether the applicant meets the evaluation criteria for obtaining particular benefits. There is no examination or cross-examination when an oral report is being given.

Written reports may be used in place of, or exclusively for, testimony or oral reporting. The written report is generally the only type of report required by the insurance adjustor for settling claims. Regardless of any testimony or oral reporting, a written report is issued to the referring party in almost all cases. Rarely will a party request that a written report not be submitted.

REFERENCES

Anderson, R. H. Vocational Expert Testimony: "The New Frontier for the Rehabilitation Professional," *Journal of Rehabilitation* 45 (1979):39,40,74.

DeMaio-Feldman, D. "The Occupational Therapist as an Expert Witness." *American Journal of Occupational Therapy* 41 (1987):591–4.

Jackson, T. P. L. "Presenting Expert Testimony," *Trail* 11 (1975): 41–3.

Osterweis, M., Kleinman, A. and Mechanic, (eds). *Pain and Disability: Clinical, Behavioral and Public Policy Perspectives*. Washington, DC: National Academy Press, 1987.

Smith, S. L. "The Forensic Model of Occupational Therapy." *Occupational Therapy in Health Care* Vol 1 (Winter 1985/86): 17–22.

CHAPTER SEVEN

THE PHYSICAL CAPACITIES EVALUATION IN THE EDUCATIONAL MODEL

PREVOCATIONAL EVALUATION SEES MOST USE IN the educational model of practice. The vocational evaluator and the work adjustment specialist compliment the occupational therapist on offering services. Vocational services focus primarily on assessing actual and potential skills and knowledge, but also deal with assessing and developing appropriate work benefits. Occupational therapists assess prevocational skills, including the patient's fine and gross motor abilities to meet the physical demands of work and the need for adapting tools, techniques, environments, and cognitive abilities to the job. They also offer counsel regarding preventive health and occupational care and intervene for remediation in the areas they have evaluated for readiness.

Public law 94-142, the Education for All Children Act, mandates occupational therapy as an educational profession as well as a medical profession (Gilfoyle 1984). The needs of special education students include both therapeutic-related services as well as academics. Often, experiential learning is incidental to the special education student's curriculum. Therefore, occupational therapy intervention for these students may well include an assessment of hand and cognitive skills as well as an assessment of gross motor abilities to meet the physical demands of work.

The public school student fits into the educational model as well. With today's emphasis on moving both emotionally disturbed and mentally retarded individuals from institutions to less restrictive group homes and other transitional living arrangements, many of these individuals are receiving Title XIX funding. The regulations for Title XIX intermediate care facilities include active treatment with, as much as possible, a goal of normalization. Thus. the services offered in group homes focus not only on ac-

tivities of daily living, but also on employment. Likewise, agencies with transitional living programs for individuals with brain injuries and others with handicaps may be clients of a state's vocational rehabilitation services agency.

Adult day care centers are becoming more prevalent, and along with them comes the need for returning their clientele to the mainstream of life. Whether a given individual has a mental health, neurological or developmental disorder, or is merely aged, work activity is a consideration in his or her return to functionality in daily life. This work may be at the volunteer level, or it may be supportive or competitive work. In either case, there is potential for intervention by occupational therapy.

REFERRAL SERVICES

Individual Education Plan Team

The individual education plan (IEP) team provides services for the special education student. The IEP, mandated by public law 94-142, outlines short- and long-term educational and related goals for the student's curriculum. Specifically, it(1) sets out academic achievement goals for the student and (2) establishes special education and related therapeutic services which must be provided to assist the student in meeting the academic goals identified (Figure 1).

When a student approaches 21 years of age, the curriculum involves preparing the student for adult life, including employment. Occupational therapists then offer services for both evaluation and remediation of fine- and gross-motor abilities, as well as functional abilities. Consequently, when the IEP team identifies a vocational learning objective, it may be to develop work tolerance or assess physical capacities, or both. Occupational therapy is the discipline that primarily addresses this objective. Direct services may be established services supplemented by teacher and parent follow-up or consultation.

Individual Habilitation Plan Team

Like the IEP services team, the individual habilitation plan (IHP) team sets learning objectives. Unlike the IEP, however, the scope of the plan is not limited to education, but reflects all spheres of life: home, work, community, and personal care. The physical capacities evaluation may be beneficial in identifying the resident's ability to meet the physical demands of a job, leisure interests, or therapeutic fitness programs.

Most certification and accreditation standards, such as Title XIX, require annual evaluations of residents in both community homes and institutions. The therapist who is a member of the IHP team has the opportunity to affect what goes into the IHP. The therapist is able to identify work-related services that are beneficial to the resident. The occupational therapist has an obligation to evaluate the resident as to whether he or she is capable of receiving each service the discipline offers.

General Service Plan Team

When more than one agency coordinates services for a resident's therapy and training, the services will be identified and set by the ISP team. This type of collaborative plan is often referred to as a generic or general service plan (GSP). The GSP team oversees and plans programs for the broad overall activity in the resident's life (Figure 2).

Here again, the therapist or GSP team has the obligation to identify services that address the resident's needs based upon the evaluation's findings. If the various agencies bring to light the need for services that have not been previously identified, these services need to be incorporated in the GSP. Among the services the therapist provides are work-related services for which physical capacities evaluation may be used to establish baseline, as well as progress, data.

General Considerations in Referrals

Once any one of the IEP, IHP, and GSP has been developed, it becomes the overall service plan, incorporating the team approach for the individual student, resident, or client. Long- and short-term goals are a part of each plan, making routine periodic evaluations necessary. This allows modification and the plan is thus flexible, accommodating itself to the individual's needs and progress. The therapist's services are offered primarily on two levels: direct or consultative.

When only consultative services are called for, the people responsible for implementing the services receive in-service training and carry out the routine therapeutic plan. The therapist then reviews the progress at least monthly and, if necessary, modifies, reaffirms, or discontinues the treatment program. When an individual has reached a specific goal, the program relating to that goal is terminated.

In the education model more than in other models, the therapist must be aggressive in securing physician referral for evaluation and treatment. This is because the physician frequently plays a less dominant role than in the other models of practice. Consequently, the therapist must ensure that there is a mechanism for the physician referral when such referral is necessary under licensing law or other policies. A medical director may be responsible for reviewing and signing the entire plan, and this, in general, constitutes the physician's referral. However, a medical director rarely is directly involved with the therapy, and other means generally are needed to secure a specific referral.

INDICATION FOR PREVOCATIONAL SERVICES

The needs of the adolescent and young adult public school student are largely prevocational. The therapist in the school system directs the therapeutic programming as one of the comprehensive services offered to the student. Along with the teacher, the occupational therapist and possibly the physical therapist, vocational evaluator, and other related specialists assist the student in finding employment upon leaving school. Foundational skills, particularly those related to the student's being able to meet the physical demands of work, are assessed by instruments such as a physical capacities evaluation, hand function evaluation, or perceptual evaluation. In evaluating physical capacities and hand function, it is important to assess the developmental level of pinching and grasping patterns, as well as the overall levels of integration of pathological reflexes and their residual effect on posture, body mechanics, and general functional capabilities. It may not always be possible to fully remedy these developmental lags, but adaptive techniques should be taught to enhance functional abilities as much as is feasible.

Prevocational services can be given to clients in out-patient service facilities. Frequently, these facilities include mental health centers. Often, the foundational skills needed for vocational endeavors are weak or absent in clients with a mental health problem. Conditions may sometimes be identified by administering a physical capacities evaluation. General physical reconditioning is frequently required, and preventive measures and side effects from medication must be addressed. Deficits in sensory integration, slow developmental progress, perceptual disabilities, behavioral rituals, and fears all contribute to a client's lacking the foundational skills for vocational readiness. For this population, occupational therapy, the physical capacities evaluation, and work related services are crucial.

Occupational therapy intervention at the prevocational level focuses on preparing the student for accepting vocational services and ultimately mainstreaming in all areas of life. The services are directed toward increasing the individual's likelihood of obtaining competitive employment and entering into a lifestyle that more and more offers opportunities for interacting with nonhandicapped persons. The therapist intervenes to assist the individual in taking advantage of the opportunities. Evaluation and remediation both are important at this level. Remediation may include not only developing the individual's physical capacities, but also adapting the environment, tools, and tasks to the individual.

Vocational evaluators are new members of the educational team and are beginning to work collaboratively with adolescent and young adult public school special education students. Students needing therapy are being identified in their early adolescence so that vocational counselors may track their progress throughout the school program. In this way, therapists are able to provide vocational consultation as well as establish a relationship with the student. Sometimes the relationship continues after the student completes the school program and even on into the time he or she begins self-supportive employment.

VOCATIONAL SERVICES

Community-based vocational programs have a wide range of services for clients. In these programs, the emphasis is on mainstreaming the client into all spheres of community life. The therapist's services may span both the work and home environments of the client's daily life. The therapist should work closely with the other vocational specialists, giving both consultation and direct services. The latter may include evaluation, training, and job placement, maintenance, and advancement. The work involved may be sheltered, modified, supported, or competitive.

In the community based situations, the occupational therapist's services are directed toward evaluating whether a specific job is appropriate for a particular resident or client. Intervention is either to remedy a problem, such as inadequate strength, or overcome a barrier by adaptation. This is a growing area for therapists. Given the current trend toward deinstitutionalization and preparing the handicapped for work following school, as well as the attention that is beginning to be paid to the elderly population that is in good health, community-based services are a growing area for therapists who desire to work within the confines of the educational model.

REFERENCES

Gilfoyle, E. M. "Transformation of a Profession." *American Journal of Occupational Therapy* 38 (1984):575–84.

Langdon, H. G., and Langdon, L. D. *Initiating Occupational Therapy Programs within the Public School System: A Guide for Occupational Therapists and Administrators.* Thorofare, NJ: Charles B. Slack, 1983.

88

INDIVIDUALIZED EDUCATION PROGRAM
LOUISIANA DEPARTMENT OF EDUCATION

Instructional Plan   Page 2 of 5   System ABC Parish School System   Student Name Kent Jones
Meeting Date(s) 08/25/87   DOB 06/11/67   ID #

GENERAL STUDENT INFORMATION   Upon completing school Kent has a vocational objective of light material handling in a competitive job. It appears he will initially have a job coach.

SPECIAL EDUCATIONAL CURRICULUM NEEDS

RELATED SERVICE(S) NEEDS   Occupational Therapy

CURRICULUM AREA   Motor

CURRICULUM AREA

CURRENT PERFORMANCE Bilateral hand strength approximately 15 psi. Able to handle weights up to 15-20 lbs. on an occasional basis with limited safety.

CURRENT PERFORMANCE

ANNUAL GOAL

Method of Measurement   Physical Capacities Evaluation (including hand strength dynomometer testing)

Date Achieved

Method of Measurement

ANNUAL GOAL Increase hand strength by 10 psi bilaterally; Increase general strength to frequently & safely handle up to 25 lbs.

SHORT-TERM OBJECTIVES (Number each objective. Include conditions and evaluation criteria.)	Dates Achieved
CODE THE STUDENT WILL BE ABLE TO:	
M1 Progressively increase hand strength by approximately 1 psi per month.	
M2 Learn good body mechanics for safe handling of weights.	
M3 Increase general strength with pro- gressively improved endurance.	

PERSONNEL RESPONSIBLE

SHORT-TERM OBJECTIVES (Number each objective. Include conditions and evaluation criteria.)	Dates Achieved
CODE THE STUDENT WILL BE ABLE TO:	

PERSONNEL RESPONSIBLE

Reprinted with permission from the Louisiana Department of Education.

Figure 1 Individual education program (IEP). This plan is mandated by the Louisiana Department of Education and is developed by the special education teacher in consultation with specialists from related disciplines.

GENERAL SERVICE PLAN

GENERAL SERVICE COMPONENT

Date: _____ May 29, 1986

Casemanager: _____ Smith

FOR

Charles

_____

Summary of Evaluative Data	Long Range Goals	Service Needs	Service Availability	Person & Agency Responsible for Obtaining Service	Service Initiation Date	Anticipated Service Duration	Evaluation Procedure	Review Schedule
Numerous as well as out-of-state institutionalizations. Placed in community Group Home 2/22/84	Normalized environment in less restrictive setting	Community Group Home	Yes	XYZ Agency 1 Main Street New Orleans, LA Joan White, Home Manager	5/30/86	Ongoing	Review all evaluative data on client's progress and revise GSP as needed	Once a year thru GSP
Structural program to develop prevocational skills	To work at least 20 hours a week in the community with non-handicapped peers	Day Developmental Training	Yes	Enterprises, Inc. 2 Park Avenue New Orleans, LA Mary Jones, Supervisor	6/2/86	Ongoing	Review all evaluative data on client's progress and revise GSP as needed	Once a year thru GSP
Poor hand grasp for work. Unsafe mobility for independent travel.	Increase adequate hand strength; conditioning to keep head up and improve posture for safe independent travel.	Occupational Therapy	Yes	Prof. Occ. Therapy Services 2727 Houma Blvd. Metairie, LA Susan Smith, LOTR	10/28/85	Ongoing	Review all evaluative data on client's progress and revise GSP as needed	Once a year thru GSP

Figure 2 General Service Plan (GSP). This plan reflects the overall inter-agency programming for a client in a nonresidential setting.

CHAPTER EIGHT

GUIDE FOR WRITING A PHYSICAL CAPACITIES EVALUATION REPORT

VARIOUS FORMATS ARE USED FOR THE PHYSICAL capacities evaluation report in the four models of practice. A specific format may be preferred by the physician, insurance company carrier, lawyer, or vocational counselor. The therapist should acquaint the referral source with the various report formats.

A *narrative report* (usually three to six typed pages) may be necessary for lawyers and vocational counselors. When testifying in legal cases, the therapist can recall the details more clearly from a narrative report. The physician who is testifying may also refer to the therapist's narrative report for a concise review of a patient's medical care and a comprehensive report of the patient's current functional and physical status.

The narrative report includes the patient's subjective complaints, objective measurements, scores on standardized tests, and the therapist's recommendations. The report should explain the patient's abilities and restrictions in relation to work, play, and self-maintenance.

A *profile report* is usually preferred by insurance carriers and physicians. Such a report may be as brief as a one-page checklist. Frequently, an insurance carrier's own report will be sent by a physician. The physician refers the patient for a physical capacities evaluation, and the therapist fills out the insurance company's physical capacities form. A brief summary and the profile form are approved by the physician and then sent to the insurance carrier.

The therapist may prefer to develop profile forms that can be filled in with numerical measurements. This enables the therapist to perform sequential evaluations and compare the patient's test responses over time. Also, a small section for comments is often helpful in explaining the qualitative aspects of the patient's performance.

A *combination narrative and profile report* may be used for writing a physical capacities evaluation. The narrative section is shorter than a regular narrative report, usually no longer than two typed pages. The narrative part summarizes the findings and recommendations of the therapist.

The profile section in the combination report may be longer than the regular profile report. For example, in the Smith Physical Capacities Evaluation (SPCE), there are separate sections for each of the 20 physical demands. In addition, a brief narrative report is combined with the SPCE to emphasize specific details and summarize the findings.

No matter what format is used, the physical capacities evaluation report should include an assessment of several factors in each separate physical capacity evaluation. It should also include the purpose of the assessment, an analysis of the patient's performance in job-related physical demands, and an assessment of the patient's endurance, pain, fatigue, swelling, and limitations of movement. The therapist should indicate the patient's tolerance in performing each of the 20 physical demands that are required in specific activities listed in *The Dictionary of Occupational Titles*. The therapist should also make a definite statement concerning the patient's ability to return to a former job or to perform sedentary, light, medium, heavy, or very heavy work, as defined in *The Dictionary of Occupational Titles*.

SAMPLE REPORT FORMATS UTILIZED IN THE FOUR MODELS OF PRACTICE

The forms on the following pages illustrate various models of reporting. Pages 93–114 contain ex-

91

amples of profile reports and narrative reports written for use in the rehabilitation model. The combined narrative and profile reports shown on pages 115–118 are written for use in the industrial model. Combined narrative and profile reports shown on pages 119–128 are used in the legal model. Finally, the report for the educational model, pages 129–130 is unique as compared to the reports of the other three models.

HAND REHABILITATION CENTER LTD.
901 WALNUT STREET
PHILA., PA. 19107
Telephone (215) 629-0980

Surgery:
James M. Hunter, M.D.
Lawrence H. Schneider, M.D.
Scott H. Jaeger, M.D.
Marwan A. Wehbé, M.D.
Stephen L. Gish, M.D.

Hand Therapy:
Evelyn J. Mackin, LPT, Director
Anne D. Callahan, MS, OTR/L, Asst. Director
Patricia L. Baxter, OTR/L
Pamela McEntee, OTR/L
Wandra Miles, OTR/L
Melanie Ballard, OTR/L
Richard Read, R.P.T.
Barbara Goodwyn, R.P.T.
Paul Brou-Keder, R.P.T.
Susan Toth, OTR/L.
Patricia M. Byron, M.A., O.T.R.
Elaine Muntzer, R.P.T.
Laura A. Bruening, OTR./L
Susan Tribus, O.T.R./L.
Marianne Koehler, OTR./L.
Karen M. Stewart, MS, OTR./L.

Administrator
Charles W. Coombs

PHYSICAL CAPACITY EVALUATION

NAME: ███████

CHART: 28023-0

DATE: July 10, 1985

EXAMINER: ███████, OTR/L

HISTORY:

███████ is an 18-year old right handed female who sustained a hyperextension injury of her left wrist on April 15, 1984 while at work. Comprehensive rehabilitation services were provided for this patient for a period of one year and three months. Extensive medical work-up has been performed including a rheumatology study which was negative, an EMG and sensory evaluation which was negative and an arthrogram and bone scan which was negative. ███████ feels the patient's left wrist possibly has a ligamentous injury which cannot be perceived through physical examination. Swelling and tendinitis are frequent and regular in the patient's left wrist when she attempts to perform functional activities. The patient wears a futura wrist splint to support her wrist and prevent repetitive motion.

███████ reports that since the time of her injury she has experienced decreased strength and endurance in her left hand. She reported that she has difficulties sweeping, vacuuming, driving a car, and performing functional tasks at home. The purpose of this evaluation is to assess the patient's physical abilities and restrictions related to performance of work activities. This test is composed of three components including hand function measurements, administration of standardized tests and observation of performance of physical demands inherent in work activities.

HAND FUNCTION MEASUREMENTS:

Grip strength was evaluated with the Jamar Dynamometer. Grip strength measured as follows:

	RIGHT HAND	LEFT HAND
FIRST LEVEL (Tight fisted grip)	58 lbs.	18 lbs.
SECOND LEVEL	65 lbs.	21 lbs.
THIRD LEVEL	62 lbs.	20 lbs.
FOURTH LEVEL	62 lbs.	24 lbs.
FIFTH LEVEL (Extended finger grip)	64 lbs.	18 lbs.

Pinch strength was evaluated with the pinch meter. Lateral pinch, the force applied by the thumb to the side of the index finger, measured 22 lbs. for the right thumb and 19 lbs. with the left thumb. Tip pinch measured with the force applied with the tip of each finger to thumb as follows:

	RIGHT HAND	LEFT HAND
Index-thumb	22 lbs.	10 lbs.
Middle-thumb	15 lbs.	10 lbs.
Ring-thumb	9 lbs.	5 lbs.
Little-thumb	5 lbs.	4 lbs.

Three-point pinch measured the force applied by the index and middle fingers to the thumb= 20 lbs. with the right hand and 13 lbs. with the left hand.

Hand volume was recorded to measure swelling after performance of the test activities. Swelling was equal bilaterally and did not increase after performance of the task.

ADMINISTRATION OF STANDARDIZED TESTS:

The Valpar Whole Body Range of Motion Work Sample was administered to assess ███████'s ability to reach, handle and manipulate in various body postures such as reaching overhead and stooping below waist level. The patient scored in the 35th percentile which is below normal. She complained of discomfort due to the repetitive manipulation required in this work sample.

The Valpar Simulated Assembly Work Sample was administered to evaluate speed of coordination for repetitive tasks. Patti was able to score in the 70th percentile for this work sample. She was required to perform repetitive three-part assembly task on a rotating wheel for a 20 minute times test. She accomplished this task well.

OBSERVATION OF PERFORMANCE OF PHYSICAL DEMANDS INHERENT IN WORK:

This patient was observed performing repetitive physical job requirements for three hours. She demonstrated the following abilities and restrictions:

PHYSICAL TASK: Comments

Standing: This patient demonstrated no difficulty standing intermittently throughout this three hour evaluation. She did report a history of phlebitis and tendonitis in the left knee. If she works in a job that requires prolonged standing it may be necessary for her to use a stool occasionally for sitting.

Sitting: This patient did not have difficulty sitting for prolonged periods of time.

Walking: Walking tolerance is fair. She reported difficulty walking for prolonged distances due to phlebitis and left knee tendonitis.

Lifting: The patient was observed lifting and carrying maximum comfortable weight in each hand and with both hands. With the right hand she was able to lift and carry 5 lbs. maximum. With the left hand she was able to lift 2 lbs. maximum. When she used both hands she was able to lift 7½ lbs. and carry it a distance of 25 feet.

93

HAND REHABILITATION CENTER
Philadelphia, PA

PHYSICAL CAPACITIES EVALUATION/SHORT FORM

DATE: ___March 25, 1985___

PATIENT NAME: ▇▇▇▇

PATIENT NUMBER: ___29914-9___

DIAGNOSIS: ___Laceration and repair of flexor tendons of right index and middle___
___fingers and right median nerve.___

Hand Dominance: _X_ Right ___ Left ___Ambidextrous___
___Changed to R___   ___Changed to L___

Occupation: ___Cook___

HAND EVALUATION:

Maximum Grip/Pinch Strength: ___recorded on Jamar Dynamometer # 8867___
___and Pinch Meter___

Grip R _40 lbs._ Level 1 2 3 4 _5_ Key pinch R _20 lbs._ Pulp pinch R _8 lbs._

Grip L _98 lbs._ Level 1 2 _3_ 4 5 Key pinch L _28 lbs._ Pulp pinch L _15 lbs._

Joints Range of Motion/Limitations: ___Limited flexion of right index and middle___
___fingers.___

Sensibility:

Protective Sensation: R _X_ Normal _____ Impaired _____ Absent
Ability to Perceive   L _X_ Normal _____ Impaired _____ Absent
Temperature and
Painful Stimuli:

Discriminative   R _____ Normal _X_ Impaired _____ Absent
Sensation:
Ability to perceive   L _X_ Normal _____ Impaired _____ Absent
size, shapes and
textures:

Hand Restrictions: R _X_ _____ Left _____ Both

Patient can lift/carry: Mark right (R) or left (L) in appropriate box:
Maximum lbs. 5 or _5_ 10 15 20 25 30 35 40 45 50 55 60 65 70 75 80 above 80 lbs.
less

Frequently _____ _____ _____ _____ _____ _____
Occasionally _____ _____ _R_ _____ _L_ _____
Never   _____ _____ _____ _____ _____ _____

Patient can use hands to repetitive: Mark (R) or (L) for each task:
A Simple Grasping   B Pushing & Pulling   C Fine Manipulation
 _R_ L   _R_ No   _R_ L _R_   _Yes_ L _R_ No
Yes No   _Yes_ No

Released to Work: Full Duty Date: _____ Restricted Duty _X_
Comments:
Reviewed by therapist ▇▇▇▇▇▇▇▇ Date: ___March 25, 19▇▇___
Reviewed by surgeon

Pushing/Pulling:

This patient had difficulty pushing and pulling objects with her left hand. She complained of pain in her left wrist during this activity. She had no difficulty pushing or pulling objects with the right hand.

Reaching:

No difficulty observed.

Handling:

This patient can handle light weight objects without difficulty. She did experience discomfort, fatigue and pain when she attempted to lift heavy objects weighing over 2 lbs.

Manipulating:

This patient was able to manipulate objects rapidly with either her right or left hands. She did complain of some discomfort in her left wrist after she had performed repetitive manipulation with her left hand for 2 hours.

SUMMARY AND RECOMMENDATIONS:

The purpose of this Physical Capacity Evaluation is to determine the patient's physical abilities and restrictions to perform her former job. The job description of hostess was supplied by the Marriott Corporation for analysis prior to this test. This patient was evaluated for her potential to perform this work and it was noted that she was able to perform the task of greeting customers, selling, exhibiting pleasant personality, and informing manager of any situation requiring attention. Based on her performance, it appears that she would have great difficulty performing repetitive cleaning of tables and booths, cleaning of glass and doors, cleaning bathrooms, refilling the salad bar with food and condiments and preparing the food with tomato slicers and food processors. She is unable to perform her former job due to difficulty with lifting, carrying, pushing, pulling, and handling objects weighing over 1 lb. with her left hand.

It is noted that this patient has the physical abilities to perform standing, sitting, reaching, handling, and manipulating of light weight objects. Therefore, it is suggested that this patient be placed in a job as cashier.

▇▇▇▇▇▇ _OTR/L_
▇▇▇▇▇▇

PB:mjp

94

PROFESSIONAL OCCUPATIONAL THERAPY SERVICES

2727 HOUMA BOULEVARD —— TELEPHONE 504/455-7093

METAIRIE, LOUISIANA 70006

SUSAN L. SMITH, M.A., L.O.T.R., F.A.O.T.A.
DIRECTOR

BARBARA C. LEBLANC, MED., L.O.T.R.
STAFF

****
06/04/91

FUNCTIONAL EVALUATION

Mr. ********, a 45 year old man, had been referred for a Functional Evaluation. Upon his arrival obvious signs of disability were observed as the client walked with a cane. However he showed no obvious sign of disfigurement. The client had driven from his home in Patterson, Mississippi. Throughout the three hour evaluation Mr. ******** gave his full cooperation and sincere efforts to all that was asked of him.

The Functional Evaluation consists of three components. These are as follows.

1. Review of Medical Documentation: This review is done in order for the therapist to learn of the client's pathology, any medical contra-indications there might be for activity, and medical prognosis.

2. Activity Interview: The activity interview ascertains the client's general life style level of activity and post injury level of activity. Topics covered are work history, educational background, family and home responsibilities, leisure time interests, and capabilities for personal care.

3. Performance Component: This assessment is selected depending upon what residual problems the client exhibits. As the client's condition affects his whole body functioning, the Smith Physical Capacities Evaluation was chosen for this portion. This assessment measures the way a person utilizes their body as a whole in being able to meet the physical demands of activity.

ACTIVITY INTERVIEW:

Mr. ******** states that he is a high school graduate. All other job skills have been learned through on the job training. He states that he has no further formal training or advanced education.

The client related that he began his career life in the U.S. Army. Here he states that his MOS was aircraft mechanic. However he states that he did no mechanical work. Since discharged from the Army in 1963 he has worked as a construction laborer in various jobs. He states that he has found that he has been unable to work since the time of his injury in the Fall of 1990.

The client states that he is separated and lives alone in a mobile home. He related that he is able to manage his household activities of cooking, shopping, laundry, and cleaning for himself. However he states that he can do none of these activities fully. The client states that he would usually have a garden about 15 feet long and with 15 to 20 rows of vegetables. However he found that he could not manage this this year and consequently only planted four rows. He is managing this.

In his leisure time the client states that he has had a few interests throughout his life. He enjoys gardening, fishing from off the shore, and a little reading. He is no longer able to fish and has had to limit his gardening. However he continues to be able to read.

The client has a car with an automatic transmission, power brakes and steering. He related that he develops pain in his left leg when driving even only a short distance. Consequently he limits his driving to local driving. That is except for driving to appointments outside of the local area when absolutely necessary. However he attempts to find someone who would drive him for any out of town needs. He states that today he was unable to find anyone to drive him. Consequently, he stated that he came to the city last night. He stated that he drove at a slow pace and it took him about four and a half to five hours to make the trip. He was planning to drive back to Patterson after this evaluation. His maximum relatively comfortable period is about an hour of driving.

In his personal care activities of dressing, bathing, grooming, and feeding the client related that he continues to be independent. He proceeds at his own pace and has adapted some of his methods. He states that at times when he is in the bathtub, if he lays down, he may get a "catch" in his neck and must stay in the position until it resolves.

PERFORMANCE COMPONENT:

On the Physical Capacity Evluation Mr. ******** showed himself to be extremely limited in his ability to meet the physical demands of activity. He was dependent upon a cane or other external support for any activity which he was doing on his feet. Those activities which necessitated hip flexion, i.e. walking, climbing, lifting from the low plane, turning with spinal rotation, and sitting all caused the client to have varying degrees of discomfort in his left hip and thigh. Also activities which placed a pressure on the left hip caused him discomfort in that hip, i.e. left side lying. Other activities, pushing, and push-pulling caused him to have some low back discomfort. Also, some upper right back discomfort was experienced when doing activities of reaching across his body with his right hand. Therefore his endurance for activity was seen to be a definite factor in limiting his function. As well the client tends to attempt to keep his weight bearing off his left foot his spontaneity of movement and agility is very much limited.

It was seen that Mr. ******** is realistically able to handle weights, only on an occasional basis, of up to 10 pounds. In the low and overhead planes the amount is substantially less. The client has limited functional standing and sitting endurance. His left hand grasp is considerably below the mean for men in his age range relative to strength of grasp.

For details of Mr. ********' performance on the Physical Capacity Evaluation please see that portion of this report.

MEDICAL DOCUMENTATION:

This therapist has for review several medical documents. They include the following:

1. What appears to be physician visit notes dating from 08-23-90 throughout 11-27-90. This is unsigned.

2. Report by Joseph F. Guenther, M.D. (Family Medicine) dated October 4, 1990.

1. Orthopeadic Evaluation specifically of the left hip to determine if there has developed a concern with the client's prosthesis.

2. Evaluation by a rheumotologist relative to the client's degenerative arthritic concerns.

3. Evaluation by a physical therapist for postural and gait concerns.

In summary, Mr. ******* is a man in his mid career years. At this time he cannot meet the physical demands for work. At this time there does not appear to be any further medical or surgical intervention recommended. However it is this therapist's opinion that further medical and rehabilitation evaluation should be conducted. If in the future Mr. ******* can get relief of his discomfort and ability to be free of external devices and a more normal weight bearing pattern he may be able to return to some type of work. It would depend upon the degree of relief he is able to get whether he will be able to return to the competitive labor market. Therefore, it is seen that the scope of job opportunities which have now been closed and may only be ******* in the past have now been closed and may only be narrowly opened in the future or they may remain closed.

Susan L. Smith, LOTR

---

3. Orthopeadic Evaluation by Robert T. Van Uden, Jr., M.D., dated December 14, 1990.

4. Orthopeadic Evaluation by Gerard L. Murtagh, M.D., dated December 12, 1990.

5. Report by E.E. Robinson, III, M.D., of a neurosurgical evaluation dated January 7, 1991.

The diagnostic impression of Dr. Guenther in his report of October 4, 1990 was:

1. Cervical Strain
2. Lumbar Strain
3. Thoracic Strain
4. Status-Post Left Hip Replacement

Dr. Guenther recommends a course of conservative home and office therapy.

In Dr. Murtagh's report of December 12, 1990 he states that x-rays demonstrate degenerative arthritis involving the lumbar spine. His clinical impression is:

1. Cervical Contusion and Strain
2. Lumbar Strain and Contusion
3. Strain of the Left Hip

Also in this report Dr. Murtagh states that on x-rays there is a evidence of total hip prosthesis with some questionable loosening.

Dr. Van Uden states that x-ray findings of the cervical and lumbar spine as well as MR Scan of the cervical and lumbar spine reveal some degenerative changes. However he does not find any other orthopeadic problem. He refers Mr. ******* for a neurosurgical evaluation by Dr. Robinson. Dr. Robinson does not find evidence of neurological deficits.

OPINION:

Mr. ******* is a man in his mid career years. He has worked throughout his career life as a laborer. In 1977 it is reported that the client had a left total hip replacement. He returned to work and worked until the time of his recent injury, which he reported was in the Fall of 1990. At this time Mr. ******* cannot meet the physical demands for any work. Even sedentary work he would have difficulty in being able to tolerate any long sitting. Unless Mr. ******* can have substantial relief of the discomfort particularly in his left thigh and hip he cannot be anticipated to be able to return to the competitive labor market.

In the medical documentation which this therapist has for review there is no current indications for medical or surgical intervention. It is seen that Mr. ******* has a non-prescribed cane, which he is using consistently. This does not allow him optimal mechanical advantage of the cane. As well it is placing a disproportionate mechanical force on other joints in his body. This not only limited to his cane but the fact that he does not put an equal weight bearing on both his feet. As there is some indication that the client's prosthesis may be loosening, and the fact that he has evidence of degenerative arthritis, it is this therapist's opinion that he should have further specialty medical and therapy evaluation with possible followup treatment. The

96

Professional Occupational Therapy Services, Inc.
2727 Houma Boulevard
Metairie, Louisiana 70006

Name:

Date: 06/04/91

SMITH PHYSICAL CAPACITIES EVALUATION

This evaluation is designed to measure the gross function capacities and limitations of a person. It is based upon the 20 broad physical demands which the U.S. Department of Labor utilizes in specifying the primary requisite physical demands for jobs in the national competitive labor market.

The evaluation is rated using the following rating scale. The standard of measure being a cross-section of persons of the same age range and sex as the person being evaluated.

Within Normal Range (WNR); Fair; Poor; Unable

Walking:

Request:
1. To walk normally 100 yards on level surface, turning to reverse direction at least one (1) time.

Performance:
a. Type of gait: Fair
b. Appliances Used: Non-Prescribed Single
                        Point Cane
c. Endurance: Fair-
d. Safety: Within Normal Range-
e. Ability to turn: Fair

2. The client's estimate of distance and length of time they are able to walk.

Estimate:
a. Distance inside: Up to around a supermarket
b. Distance outside: Up to two blocks
c. Time inside: Up to 15 minutes
d. Time outside: Up to 15 minutes

COMMENT: Walking required in client's job. The client used his cane in his right hand. He walked at a moderately slow place with moderate dependence upon the cane. He developed some soreness in his left thigh. He stopped to turn rather than make an agile turn. The client's estimates of times and distances he is able to walk are those which he states that he is able to do in his daily life. He remarked that he felt that soon he would need crutches.

Running:

Request: To run 30 yards on a level surface turning to reverse direction at least one (1) time.

Performance:
a. Ability: Unable
b. Endurance:
c. Type of gait:
d. Safety:

COMMENT: Running required in emergency situations in client's job only. The client is unable to run due to his lack of standing/walking balance and inability to toe-off.

Jumping:

Request: To jump from an 18", and then a 30" high platform onto a level surface, landing on both feet.

Performance:
a. Ability: 18": Not Tested   30":Not Tested
b. Balance: 18":   30":
c. Safety: 18":   30":
d. Endurance: 18":   30":

COMMENT: Jumping required in client's job. Jumping was not tested as a medical precaution relative to the client's left hip problem.

97

4. Straight Ladder (8', 11" rise):
   To climb up and down five (5) consecutive times.

Performance:
a. Foot-over-foot: X
   Foot-by-foot: X
b. Hand-over-hand:
   Hand-on-rail:
   Hand-by-hand:
c. Balance: Fair
d. Safety: Fair-
e. Endurance: Fair+
f. Ability: Poor

5. Step Ladder (5', 12" rise): To climb up and down once carrying a 10 pound pail in the hand of client's choice.

Performance:
a. Foot-over-foot:
   Foot-by-foot: X
b. Balance: Fair-
c. Safety: Within Normal Range-
d. Endurance: Within Normal Range-
e. Appliances Used: Non-Prescribed Single Point Cane

COMMENT: Climbing required in client's job. When ramp climbing the client used his cane in his right hand. When turning he used the rail for support. He developed left thigh soreness. This progressed in intensity. When stair climbing the client had some slight imbalance. When ascending he used the rail in his right hand and his cane in his left. When descending he used the cane in his right hand and the rail in his left. He developed some left thigh discomfort with the activity. When ascending the 6" curb the client led with his left foot and when descending with his right. At the 12" height he ascended leading with his right and as well as descending with his right. At the 18" height he ascended leading with his right and descended leading with his left. He was cautious at all times to maintain his balance. When turning the client had some slight discomfort develop in his left thigh. When straight ladder climbing the client took his primary weight on his right foot. He was unable to climb more than two rungs due to his inability to manage weight shifting onto his left foot. He depended heavily upon his hands and arms for support. He had no increase in discomfort. When step ladder climbing the client avoided weight bearing on his left foot. He used his cane in his right hand. He then stepped up the first step leading with his right foot. He was unable to manage any further climbing. He reached over the top of the ladder and placed the pail on the shelf. He then reversed his procedure in descending.

Climbing:
Request:
1. Ramp (8' x 12 degrees): To walk up and down five (5) consecutive times.

Performance:
a. Gait: Fair
b. Endurance: Fair-
c. Use of Appliances: Non-Prescribed Single Point Cane
d. Use of Handrail: None

2. Stairs (5 steps, 6" rise, wooden tread): To walk up and down two (2) consecutive times.

Performance:
a. Safety: Within Normal Range-
b. Endurance: Fair-
c. Speed: Fair
d. Use of Handrail: Up and Down
e. Use of appliances: Non-Prescribed Single Point Cane
f. Foot-over-foot: X
   Foot-by-foot:

3. Curbs (6", 12", and 18" high): To ascend and descend curbs once.

Performance:
a. Ability:
   6": Fair
   12": Fair
   18": Fair
b. Safety:
   6": Within Normal Range-
   12": Within Normal Range-
   18": Within Normal Range-
c. Appliances Used:
   6": Non-Prescribed Single Point Cane
   12": Non-Prescribed Single Point Cane
   18": Non-Prescribed Single Point Cane
d. Use of handrail:
   6": None
   12": Down
   18": Down

SMITH PHYSICAL CAPACITIES
EVALUATION - Page 5

Name: _____

Date: _____06/04/91

Crouching:
Request: To work in a squatted position for three (3)
minutes, alternating placing two pound cans (4" x 8") from
the floor to an 12" high shelf.

Performance:
a. Ability to assume position: Not Tested
b. Ability to carry out task:
c. Ability to regain standing:
d. Balance:
e. Endurance:

COMMENT: Crouching occasionally required in client's job.
Crouching not tested as medically contra-indicated by the
client's physician.

Lifting:
Request:
1. Right Hand: To alternately lift maximum weight in a
pail from a waist-high surface to floor and back five
(5) consecutive times.

Performance:
a. Number of Pounds: 20
b. Ability: Fair
c. Balance: Fair-
d. Endurance: Within Normal Range
e. Ability to grasp: Within Normal Range

2. Left Hand: To repeat (1) using the left hand.

Performance:
a. Number of Pounds: 20
b. Ability: Fair
c. Balance: Fair-
d. Endurance: Fair+
e. Ability to grasp: Within Normal Range

3. Both Hands: To alternately lift maximum weight in a
box from a waist high surface to floor five (5)
consecutive times.

Performance:
a. Number of Pounds: 15
b. Ability: Fair-
c. Balance: Fair
d. Endurance: Fair
e. Ability to grasp: Right: WNR   Left: WNR

SMITH PHYSICAL CAPACITIES
EVALUATION - Page 6

Name: _____

Date: _____06/04/91

COMMENT: Lifting of weights up to 45 to 60 pounds required
in client's job. When lifting with the right hand the client
stood directly facing the shelf using his opposite hand for
support on the shelf. He had no weight bearing on his left foot,
keeping it off the floor. He had no change in his comfort level.
When lifting with the left hand he stood with his left side to
the shelf and using his cane in his right hand for very
significant support. He had his left foot touching the floor but
with minimal weight bearing. With the activity he had a slight
increase in left thigh discomfort. When lifting with two hands
the client stood with his right side to the shelf. He stood with
his full weight bearing on his right foot and his left off the
floor. He had limited control of the box at any time but managed
the five lifts. Upon completing the two handed lifting and
standing momentarily the client had some slight increase in
discomfort in his left thigh.

Carrying:
Request: To bimanually carry the maximum weight in a box
25 yards, while walking on a level surface. The box taken
from, and returned to, a waist-high surface.

Performance:
a. Number of pounds: 4
b. Ability: Poor+
c. Balance: Fair
d. Endurance: Fair-
e. Type of gait: Fair-
f. Ability to grasp: Right: WNR   Left: WNR

COMMENT: Carrying of weights up to 45 to 60 pounds for
distances of up to 60 to 100 feet required in client's job. The
client used his cane in his right hand, holding the box handle
with only his fingers supporting it. He walked at a moderate
pace with a significant limp. As he walked he had a weakness and
soreness develop in his left knee.

99

100

SMITH PHYSICAL CAPACITIES
EVALUATION - Page 7

Name:_

Date: 06/04/91

Pushing: Push-Pull:
Request:
1. To push a wheelbarrow (heavy duty with inflated rubber tire) for 25 yards on a level surface with the maximum load client able to handle.

Performance:
a. Ability: Poor+
b. Balance on turning: Poor+
c. Endurance: Poor+
d. Number of pounds: 0
   Number of pounds at handles: 5

2. To alternately push and pull bimanually, to arm's length, the maximum in a weighted box on a waist-high rough surface, 10 times, first from a standing and then a sitting position.

Performance:
a. Number of pounds: Standing: 45   Sitting: 50
b. Ability: Standing: Poor+ Sitting: Fair
c. Endurance: Standing: Poor Sitting: WNR-
d. Range of Motion: Back: WNR   Arms: WNR
e. Ability to Grasp: Right: WNR   Left: WNR

COMMENT: Pushing required in client's job. When pushing the wheelbarrow the client walked with a severe right limp. His pace was slow and cautious. He showed good motor planning. He was somewhat anxious as to his left knee not failing him. When standing to push the box the client stood with no weight bearing on his left foot. This he used upper body strength only and he mechanically was at a disadvantage. Consequently he accomplished the activity only by sheer determination and effort. By the time he had completed the activity he had some right hip and low back discomfort. When sitting to push the box the client kept his left leg extended and braced with his right foot. Again he was at a mechanical disadvantage and had to make a great effort to accomplish the task. He had no increase in discomfort from this activity.

SMITH PHYSICAL CAPACITIES
EVALUATION - Page 8

Name:_

Date: 06/04/91

Pulling:
Request: To alternately pull and lower, in a hand-over-hand fashion the maximum weight on a single pulley (3/4" cotton rope) 10 consecutive times.

Performance:
a. Number of pounds: 25
b. Ability: Fair
c. Balance: Within Normal Range-
d. Endurance: Within Normal Range-
e. Reach: Within Normal Range
f. Visual Monitoring: Within Normal Range
g. Ability to grasp:
   Right: Within Normal Range
   Left: Within Normal Range

COMMENT: Pulling required in client's job. The client stood with slight flexion in his hips. He used his cane for balance supporting it against his left leg in the crease of his hip. As he worked he had no significant increase or decrease in his comfort level.

Stooping:
Request: To perform for three minutes, alternately standing and stooping, while bimanually placing 2 lb. cans (4" x 8") on a 42" high shelf to the floor.

Performance:
a. Ability: Within Normal Range-
b. Endurance: Poor+
c. Ability to grasp:
   Right: Within Normal Range
   Left: Within Normal Range

COMMENT: Stooping required in client's job. The client stooped with full extension of his knees and little weight bearing on his left foot. He worked at a moderate pace. By the time he had completed 1 minute and 18 seconds he was beginning to have some discomfort in his low back. By 2 1/2 minutes this had developed into pain in his right hip which radiated to his knee. He had some slight increase in discomfort in his left thigh.

SMITH PHYSICAL CAPACITIES
EVALUATION - Page 9

Name: _____

Date: 06/04/91

Reaching:
Request:
1. Overhead: From a standing position to:
   a. Bimanually pick-up a 10 lb. box from a waist-high surface, place it on an imaginary overhead surface and then return it to the waist-high surface, one (1) time.

   b. To reach a pencil, first with right and then with left hand, at the extreme of reach at right, left and across body; and at the midline, then to reach bimanually directly in front of the body.

Performance:
   a. Ability: 10 lbs.:   Poor+
                      Small Object:
   b. Range of Motion: Right: WNR   Left: WNR
                       Back: WNR   Neck: WNR
   c. Balance: Within Normal Range
   d. Coordination: Within Normal Range
   e. Grasp: Right: WNR   Left: WNR
   f. Endurance: Fair

2. Immediate:
   a. From a standing position to bimanually reach forward and pick-up a 10 lb. box from a waist-high surface and return it to that surface.

   b. Repeat l.b. in the immediate plane with therapist holding the pencil at the various points of reach. The client is seated in a straight chair.

Performance:
   a. Ability: 10 lbs: Within Normal Range-
                      Small Object: Within Normal Range-
   b. Range of Motion: Right: WNR   Left: WNR
                       Back: WNR   Neck: WNR
   c. Balance: Within Normal Range
   d. Coordination: Within Normal Range
   e. Grasp: Right: WNR   Left: WNR
   f. Endurance: Fair

SMITH PHYSICAL CAPACITIES
EVALUATION - Page 10

Name: _____

Date: 06/04/91

3. Low: Sitting:
   a. Repeat l.b., the therapist placing the pencil on the floor, at designated points while the client sits in a straight chair, and reaches.

Performance:
   a. Ability: Fair
   b. Range of Motion: Right: WNR   Left: WNR
                       Back: Fair   Neck: WNR
   c. Balance: Within Normal Range-
   d. Coordination: Within Normal Range
   e. Grasp: Right: WNR   Left: WNR
   f. Endurance: Fair-

4. Low: Standing:
   a. Repeat l.b. the therapist placing the pencil on the floor, at the designated points, while the client stands in one position.

Performance:
   a. Ability: Fair
   b. Range of Motion: Right: WNR   Left: WNR
                       Back: WNR   Neck: WNR
   c. Balance: Within Normal Range-
   d. Coordination: Within Normal Range
   e. Grasp: Right: WNR   Left: WNR
   f. Endurance: Fair-

COMMENT: Reaching in all planes required in client's job. When reaching overhead with the 10 pound box the client had inadequate balance as he reached to the extreme and forward. When reaching to mid-line with the left hand and across his body with his right hand the client had left hip discomfort develop. When reaching in the immediate plane with both right and left hands across his body the client had some discomfort develop in his right shoulder. When reaching in the low plane from sitting the client had pain his left hip when reaching to mid line with the right hand and he was unable to reach across his body due to this pain. When reaching with his left hand he had pain develop in his left hip. This was also true when reaching with both hands. When reaching to the low plane from standing the client stooped without knee flexion. When reaching with the right hand the client had moderate discomfort develop in his left hip. This was also true when reaching with both hands. When reaching with the left hand he developed pain in his right hip.

101

Kneeling:

Request: To assume a kneeling position on the floor, keeping the back straight, and maintain the position for one minute.

Performance:
a. Ability to assume position: Fair
b. Ability to regain standing: Fair
c. Balance: Within Normal Range
d. Endurance: Fair
e. Ability: Within Normal Range-

COMMENT: Kneeling required in client's job. When assuming and regaining his position the client utilized external hand support. He used substantial support, with his right hand on his cane. When in position he took his primary weight on his right knee. With the activity the client had an increase in left pain.

Crawling:

Request: To crawl on a level floor eight feet forward and then backward with the head and shoulders low.

Performance:
a. Type of crawl:
   4-point: X
   3-point:
   Other:
b. Speed: Within Normal Range-
c. Ability: Fair+
d. Endurance: Fair-

COMMENT: Crawling required in client's job. The client was moderately cautious in this activity. He used a fairly equal weight bearing pattern on his four extremities. He developed only moderate pain in the left hip. He was pleased as he anticipated greater pain.

Reclining:

Request: To assume a backlying position on the floor. When in position turn on one side, then the other, and then face-lying. Return to standing position.

Performance:
a. Ability to:
   Assume Position: Fair
   Regain Standing: Within Normal Range
   Turn Right: Within Normal Range
   Turn Left: Fair
   Turn Face-lying: Within Normal Range
b. Comfort on:
   Right: Within Normal Range
   Left: Poor
   Face: Within Normal Range
   Back: Within Normal Range

COMMENT: Reclining occasionally required in client's job. When assuming the reclining position the client utilized bilateral external hand support. When regaining his standing he put all his weight bearing on his left leg and foot to come to standing. When turning to the left the client was very cautious in his movements. When on his left he has left hip pain.

Turning:

Request:
a. With the client standing with their right side to a waist high surface, reach and lift the maximum weight in a box from this surface by only turning the trunk. Place the box on the floor and then return it to waist-high surface only using rotation of the trunk.
b. Repeat, standing with client's left side to the waist high shelf.

Performance:
a. Ability to: Right: WNR Left: WNR-
b. Balance: Right: WNR Left: WNR
c. Endurance: Right: WNR Left: Fair-
d. Number of Pounds: 10

COMMENT: Turning required in client's job. When turning to the left the client had left hip pain.

SMITH PHYSICAL CAPACITIES
EVALUATION - Page 13

Name: _____

Date: 06/04/91

Balancing:
Request: To one-leg stand, first on the right and then the left leg, for 30 seconds each.

Performance:
a. Ability to
   gain balance: Right: WNR   Left: Not Tested
b. Endurance: Right: WNR   Left:
c. Leg Dominance: Right: X   Left:
d. Quality of Balance: Right: Poor   Left:

COMMENT: Above average balance required in client's job. When balancing on his right foot the client held his left foot barely above the floor rather than with the knee flexed to 80 to 90 degrees. Left leg standing was not tested due to the client's great anxiety and as a medical/safety precaution.

Sitting:
With what ability is the client able to get in and out of a straight-back chair? Client's estimates of how long they can sit comfortably, and with what type of posture?

Performance:
a. Ability to sit: Fair
b. Ability to rise: Fair
c. Estimated Time:
   Functional Posture: Poor+
   Non-Functional Posture: Within Normal Range-

COMMENT: Sitting not required in client's job. When sitting and rising the client uses external hand support. The client is able to sit for extended periods of time in a non-functional position. His comfortable posture is with his left leg extended and his hips only slightly flexed. That is with sitting forward in the chair and using the back for support. (Sacral sitting) When sitting in a functional posture with his left knee flexed and his sitting back in the chair he tolerates only short periods of time.

SMITH PHYSICAL CAPACITIES
EVALUATION - Page 14

Name: _____

Date: 06/04/91

Standing:
What type of posture and stance does the client exhibit? Client's estimate of time he can stand.

Performance:
a. Posture: Within Normal Range
b. Stance: Within Normal Range-
c. Estimate of Time:
   Functional Posture: Up to 5 to 10 minutes
   Non-Functional Posture: Up to 1 hour

COMMENT: Standing required in client's job. The client stands with his primary weight on his right foot. When standing he always utilizes some external support. Consequently functional standing is difficult. He must have the support of a counter or something in front of him in order to stand in a functional position. The client's tolerance is limited by left hip and knee and low back discomfort. The client states that also he is beginning to have some discomfort develop in his right hip.

Hand Grasp:
As measured with a dynamometer, the strength of the client's hand grasp.

Performance:
a. Broad Grasp: Right: Fair   Left: Poor+
b. Tight Grasp: Right: WNR-   Left: Poor+
c. Hand Dominance: Right: X   Left:

COMMENT: Good bilateral hand grasp required in client's job. The client's right hand grasp was slightly one standard deviation below the mean for men in his age range. His left hand grasp strength was seen to be approximately two and a half standard deviations below the mean for men in his age range.

Handling:
Therapist's estimate of the realistic maximum weight the client is able to handle comfortably. This includes lifting, carrying, pushing, and pulling. The estimate is based on the client's performance of these sub-tests.

a. Estimate: Up to 10 pounds
b. Frequency: Routine: Frequent: Occasional:X
c. Positions:
   Overhead: Up to 5 pounds
   Frontal: Up to 10 pounds
   Right: Up to 10 pounds
   Left: Up to 5 pounds
   Low: 0

103

RESIDENT: _____ IDT DATE 08/12/91 _____ RECORD _____

OCCUPATIONAL THERAPY EVALUATION:

In the past year **** has not had occupational therapy services. **** continues to have a high level of independence. He has wholly adequate oro-motor skills for eating. He is independent in his self-care and has a moderate level of domestic skills. Initially **** was seen for a hand strengthening program. He made gains in this program developing adequate hand strength for light daily life activity.

Today when ****'s hand strength was tested he was seen to have maintained his hand strength of 40 pounds of force in each hand. It appears that **** is using his hands for more activities in his daily life, including work activity.

Also, it was seen that **** has become more conversant and spontaneous in his conversation.

SERVICE PLAN

Defer Occupational Therapy Services.

STRENGTHS

1. Good level of independence.
2. Verbal.
3. Pleasant personality.

NEEDS

1. Continue to increase participation in a variety of daily life activities.

RECOMMENDATIONS

1. None.

JOINT RANGE OF MOTION:

TRUNK ___ Within Normal Limits ___

LOWER EXTREMITY
HIP Tight Hamstrings: Left and Right
KNEES Within Normal Limits
ANKLES Within Normal Limits

UPPER EXTREMITY
SHOULDERS Within Normal Limits
ELBOW Within Normal Limits
WRIST Within Normal Limits
FINGERS Within Normal Limits

BALANCE:
SITTING Within Normal Limits
STANDING Within Normal Limits

SENSORY Within Normal Limits

MUSCLE TONE

HYPERTONIC ___ Absent ___

HYPOTONIC ___ Absent ___

NORMAL ___ Present ___

MOTOR PLANNING Within Normal Range

PATHOLOGICAL REFLEX: ___ None ___

DEFORMITIES: ___ None ___

OCCUPATIONAL THERAPY

ASSESSMENT

1. Good level of independence in self-care abilities. _____
2. Good level of capability in domestic skills. _____
3. No significant oro-motor deficits interfering with eating. _____
4. Adequate hand strength for needs: personal and work. _____
5. _____
6. _____

RECOMMENDATIONS

1. None. _____
2. _____
3. _____
4. _____
5. _____
6. _____

PLAN

1. Defer Occupational Therapy Services with re-evaluation in one year. _____
2. _____
3. _____
4. _____
5. _____
6. _____

_____ M.D.

SUSAN L. SMITH, LOTR
07 / 11 / 91   ___/___/___

104

Document 1

HAND REHABILITATION CENTER, LTD.
901 WALNUT STREET
PHILADELPHIA, PA 19107
Telephone (215) 629-0980

PHYSICAL CAPACITY EVALUATION

Surgery:
James M. Hunter, M.D.
Lawrence H. Schneider, M.D
Stephen I. Cash, M.D.
William H. Kirkpatrick, M.D.

Administrator of Rehabilitation:
Evelyn J. Mackin, L.P.T.

Hand Therapy Staff:
Patricia Baxter Pettnila, M.S., OT.R./L.
Richard Read, R.P.T.
Patricia M. Byron, M.A., OT.R./L.
Laura A. Bruening, OT.R./L.
Susan Blackmore, M.S., OT.R./L.
Colleen Burke, P.T.A.
Patricia A. Wright, M.OT., OT.R./L.
Julie Belkin, OT.R./L., CO
Patricia Totten, OT.R./L.
Veronica Keirans, OT.R./L.
Jody Dimit, P.T.

Name:

Chart No.: 36664-1

Date: March 23, 1989

Evaluator: Patricia Baxter, M.S., OTR/L

MEDICAL HISTORY AND IDENTIFYING INFORMATION:

This 40 year-old, right-hand dominant female was employed as a teaching aide in special education at Lincoln Highschool. On November 3, 1986, the pateint reported she sustained lacerations to her right ring and little fingers while cutting foods at work. The injury resulted in contractures of the right fourth and fifth fingers. Surgery was performed on the following dates and included the following procedures:

November 18, 1987, repair of laceration.
May 18, 1987, metacarpophalangeal capsulectomy, radial and ulnar collateral ligament reconstruction, tenolysis, flexor and extensor tendons of the right ring and little finger.
December 12, 1987, arthrodesis proximal interphalangeal joints of the right ring and little fingers.
October 10, 1988, extensor tenolysis, interosseous muscle resection, extensor tenorrhaphy of the right ring finger.

The patient was followed in therapy at the Hand Rehabilitation Center. At the present time, she continues therapy. The patient has not worked since the date of injury.

The patient indicates that she is single with one child. She indicates assistance is needed in self-care and

---

Document 2

HAND REHABILITATION CENTER LTD.
901 WALNUT STREET
PHILA., PA. 19107
Telephone (215) 629-0980

PHYSICAL CAPACITY EVALUATION

Surgery:
James M. Hunter, M.D.
Lawrence H. Schneider, M.D.
Scott H. Jaeger, M.D.
Marwan A. Wehbé, M.D.
Stephen I. Cash, M.D.

Hand Therapy:
Evelyn J. Mackin, L.P.T., Director
Anne D. Callahan, O.T.R., Asst. Director
Patricia L. Baxter, O.T.R.
Pamela McEntee, O.T.R.
Wandra Miles, O.T.R.
Melanie Bulind, O.T.R.
Richard Read, L.P.T.
Barbara Goodwyn, R.P.T.
Paula Breno-Kader, R.P.T.
Susan Toth, O.T.R.
Patricia M. Byron, M.A., O.T.R.
Elaine Hunter, R.P.T.
Laura A. Bruening, O.T.R.

Administrator
Charles W. Coombs

NAME:

DATE: 3/25/85

EXAMINER: , O.T.R./L

CHART: #29914-9

HISTORY AND IDENTIFYING INFORMATION:

____ is a 23-year-old right handed cook who sustained laceration of the flexor tendons to his right index and middle finger and median nerve of the right hand on September 23, 1984. Primary repair was performed on September 24, 1984 to the flexor tendons and the median nerve. At the present time, ____ complains of numbness in the median nerve distribution of his right hand which includes his thumb, index finger, middle finger, and one half of his ring finger on the radial side. The purpose of this evaluation is to indicate the patient's physical abilities and restrictions related to performance of work activities.

Hand Function Evaluations indicate the following: strength of the right hand measured 40 pounds maximum as compared to 98 pounds in the left hand; pinch strength measured 8 pounds in the right digits as compared to 15 pounds in the left digit; Sensory function measured protective sensation (ability to feel hot and cold) in the right median nerve distribution. All other areas of the right and left hand recorded normal sensation; range of motion of the right index finger is restricted due to nerve and tendon injury.

Functionally ____ can perform gross handling and simple grasping of objects with his right and left hand. He can lift 34 pounds maximum with his right hand. He can lift 63 pounds maximum with his left and 51 pounds with both hands. He can carry this weight a distance of 25 feet safely. The patient has difficulty performing fine manipulation with his right hand. He has difficulty opening bottles, and manipulating small objects due to the sensory decrease in his right thumb, index, and middle and ring fingers.

It is recommended that ____ be evaluated for job placement. He is unable to perform his former duties as a cook due to sensory deficits in his right hand, poor manipulation ability in the right, and limited strength. He is able to use his right hand for simple grasping, pushing and pulling, lifting objects of up to 35 pounds, and repetitive manipulation that does not require speed or accuracy. The patient will continue in the therpay program at the Hand Rehabilitation Center until he is placed in an alternate job. At that time, he will be discharged from our program.

____ , O.T.R./L

home-care activities. The patient noted limitations in performance of activities of daily living, with the right hand, including: Lifting and carrying trash, using hand tools for home repair, dressing, buttoning, using eating utensils, using cooking utensils, lifting and carrying pots and pans and stacks of dishes, opening containers, toilet care, hair grooming, bathing, shopping, doing laundry, making beds, sweeping, mopping, vacuuming, opening car doors, riding, and driving.

Additional medical history reported by the patient includes: A fibroid tumor and prescription glasses necessary for eyes. The patient states she is taking Motrin, Xanax, and Elavil medication.

JOB HISTORY:

The patient was employed as a teachering aide in special education for over five years. According to the Dictionary of Occupational Titles, this job requires lifting, carrying, pushing, pulling, reaching, handling, manipulating, talking, hearing and seeing. In the Dictionary, the level of work defined in this job is light work requiring up to 10 pounds of lifting. However, the patient reported as a teacher's aide in special education. She is required to lift, push, pull, and carry children weighing up to 100 lbs.

The Physical Capacity Evaluation was ordered by Dr. [redacted] to determine the patient's physical abilities and restrictions and to determine if she can return to her former job.

The Physical Capacity Evaluation consists of three components: A hand function evaluation, administration of standarized tests, and observation of performance of physical demands in job simulation.

HAND FUNCTION EVALUATION

Grip strength taken on the Jamar Dynamometer was as follows:

Jamar Dynamometer	Right Hand	Left Hand
Level I(tight grip)	17 lbs	30 lbs
Level II	28 lbs	65 lbs
Level III	34 lbs	58 lbs
Level IV	26 lbs	50 lbs
Level V(wide grip)	20 lbs	40 lbs

Pinch strength measurements were recorded with the Pinch gauge and were as follows:

Pinch	Right Hand	Left Hand
Lateral pinch	18 lbs	15 lbs
Pinch:		
Thumb/Index	12 lbs	13 lbs
Thumb/Long	10 lbs	14 lbs
Thumb/Ring	8 lbs	8 lbs
Thumb/Little	5 lbs	7 lbs

Active range of motion measurements were recorded with a goniometer as follows:

Right Hand	Index	Long	Ring	Little
MP joint(norm 0 ext/90 flex)*	10/90	20/90	50/90	15/45
PIP (norm 0/90)	0/95	20/100	55/55fused	55/55fused
DIP (norm 0/60)	0/25	0/35	45/60	25/35

The patient lacked 1.5 cm touching the index finger to her right palm. She lacked 2.5 cm touching her long finger to her palm on the right hand. The ring finger of the right hand lacked 3.5 cm touching the palm and the little finger lacked 4.5 cm. Her right thumb and left digits all were able to touch the distal palmar crease of each palm.

Volumetric measurements taken before and after the Physical Capacity Evaluation demonstrated that there was not a significant increase in the hand volume. This indicates that the patient tolerated 3 hours of manual work without swelling occurring in either her right or left hand.

ADMINISTRATION OF STANDARIZED TESTS:

Coordination and dexterity were assessed using the Jebsen-Taylor Hand Function Test. This test measures the patient's prehension abilities for activities of daily living. The seven subtests include: turning, stacking, writing, simulated eating, manipulating small objects, lifting and placing light objects, and lifting and placing one-pound objects. The patient scored within normal limits on all seven tests with her left hand. With her right hand, she scored below normal limits on writing, stacking objects, lifting light objects, and lifting one-pound objects. She scored within normal limits with her right hand for turning over objects, picking up small objects and eating. The patient reported discomfort on the back of her right hand when she was writing due to

106

sensitivity of the scar. She also complained of discomfort in her right hand when she was using eating utensils.

The Nine-Hole Peg Test was utilized to measure finger tip dexterity. The patient scored within normal limits with her right hand and her left hand. The Box and Block Test was utilized to measure reaching and handling ability. The patient scored within normal limits with her right and left hands.

OBSERVATION OF PERFORMANCE OF PHYSICAL DEMANDS OF WORK:

1) Lifting/Carrying
The patient was able to lift and carry 11 pounds with her right arm and 18 pounds with her left arm, holding a bucket at waist height over a distance of 25 feet. She was able to lift and carry 11 pounds with both arms, holding a box at waist height. She was able to lift a 7 pound dumbell with her right hand from floor level to waist height. With her left hand, she could lift a 25 pound dumbell from floor level to waist height.

2) Pushing/Pulling
The patient was able to push and pull a weighted box with 24 pounds of weight with her right hand. With her left hand, she was able to push and pull 38 pounds.

3) Reaching
The patient was able to reach overhead, forward and to floor level with her right hand without difficulty.

4) Grasping/Handling
The patient can use her right hand for grasping and handling of light, small and heavy sized objects up to 7 pounds with difficulty. She can utilize her left hand for grasping and handling of small, light and heavy sized objects weighing up to 25 pounds without difficulty.

5) Manipulation
Fine manipulation was below normal limits in the right hand for writing, stacking objects and lifting objects. Right and left hand coordination was within normal limits for fine fingertip dexterity and handling.

6) Standing, Sitting and Walking
The patient reported her standing, sitting, and walking within normal limits. She is able to perform these physical demands for eight hours with intermittent

breaks. No abnormal body posture or gait was observed during this evaluation.

7) Climbing Stairs
The patient was able to climb stairs. However, she reports that she experiences fatigue in her legs when climbing stairs, especially her right leg.

8) Kneeling, Crouching and Stooping.
The patient was able to kneel, crouch and stoop without difficulty.

9) Endurance
Endurance was tested using the Work Simulator. It is a computerized evaluation instrument that can measure the amount of power emitted by the hands and arms with a variety of tools. The test compares tool use between hands for a two minute time period. With the tool that simulates gripping of pliers, her left hand demonstrated 57% greater endurance than her right hand. her left hand demonstrated 3% greater endurance than her right hand on the tool that simulates pushing or pulling long lever arm, such as mops or brooms.

10) Sequential Testing
Sequential testing was performed on the Work Simulator. According to the research of Vermette and Berlin (1985), on sequential tests, the coefficient of variance should be less than 12% for adult males and less than 15% for adult females. The patient scored a coefficient of variance of 11.5% with her right hand and 3.5% with her left hand. This indicates that she performed consistently throughout this examination.

Grip strength was measured sequentially on the Jamar Dynamometer. According to the research of Bechtol (1954), the coefficient of variance on sequential grip test should be less than 10%. The patient scored 4.4% with her right hand and 2.6% with her left hand. This indicates consistent performance on sequential testing with both hands.

SUMMARY AND RECOMMENDATIONS:

This 40 year-old right hand dominant teaching aide sustained lacerations of her right ring and little fingers resulting in contractures on November 3, 1986. She underwent four surgical procedures and therapy. At the present time, her major difficulties with her right hand include: limited strength, frequent aching, coldness of the

107

RE: ███████   -6-   03/23/89

right hand, abnormal sweating, stiffness, muscle spasms, tingling and numbness in the right fourth and fifth fingers. Test results indicate the patient's maximum grip strength of her right hand measured 34 pounds compared to 65 pounds in the left hand. Lateral pinch measured 18 pounds in the right thumb and 15 pounds in the left thumb. Tip pinch measured 12 pounds in the right index finger and 13 pounds in the left index finger. Range of motion was restricted in the right fingers. There was no swelling during the evaluation in either hand.

The patient demonstrated the physical ability to lift 11 pounds with her right hand and 18 pounds with her left hand when carrying a bucket. When lifting dumbells, she was able to lift 7 pounds with her right hand and 25 pounds with her left hand. When carrying weight in a box, she was able to lift 11 pounds maximum. The patient was able to push and pull 24 pounds with her rigth hand and 38 pounds with her left hand. Coordination was slightly below normal limits in the right hand. The patient is able to reach, grasp and handle objects with both hands. She does experience difficulty handling objects which are large or heavy with her right hand due to limited extension of the right ring and little fingers and decreased strength of the right hand.

In summary, this patient has regained function in her right hand adequate for performance of teaching aide duties in an elementary or secondary school classroom. However, she cannot work in a special education classroom as she cannot perform the necessary lifting, carrying, pushing, and pulling required for student transfers. It is recommended that this patient be released to return to work if she can transfer as a teaching aide into a classroom that does not require lifting of over 10 pounds with her right hand.

PB/pc
████ (dt: 3/28/89)

108

HAND REHABILITATION CENTER, LTD.

901 WALNUT STREET
PHILA, PA 19107
Telephone (215) 629-0980

Surgery:
James M Hunter M.D.
Lawrence H. Schneider, M.D.
Scott H. Jaeger, M.D.
Stephen L. Cash, M.D.

Administrator of Rehabilitation
Evelyn J. Mackin, LPT.

Controller
Bruce P. Cox, CPA

Hand Therapy Staff
Barbara Goodwine Smith, RPT
Laura A. Baxter, OTR/L
Anne D. Callahan, M.S., OTR/L
Richard Read, RPT
Paula Brome Kader, RPT
Susan Toth, OTR/L
Patricia M. Byron, M.A., OTR/L
Laura A. Bruening, OTR/L
Susan Tribuzi, OTR/L
Marianne Koehler, OTR/L
Karen M. Stewart, MS., OTR/L
Gwendolyn van Strien, RPT.
Frank Angiolillo, RPT.
Gisele Larose, OTR/L
Susan Blackmore, OTR/L
Barbara L. Reeder, OTR/L
Debra Beaulieu, OTR/L

PHYSICAL CAPACITY EVALUATION

NAME: ▮▮▮▮▮ OTR/L

CHART: #31458-3

DATE: June 10, 1986

EVALUATOR: ▮▮▮▮▮ OTR/L

MEDICAL HISTORY AND IDENTIFYING INFORMATION:

This 52 year-old right hand dominant female was employed as a nurse's aide at ▮▮▮▮▮. On July 4, 1984, the patient Ms. ▮▮▮ injured her left hand on a bed while working. The patient also noted a cumulative onset of bilateral hand pain and triggering of the thumb over a period of her years of employment as a nurse's aide. Ms. ▮▮▮ did return to work since the date of injury in July, 1984, but sustained a hairline fracture of her left clavicle approximately six months later. She has not returned to work since that time. Ms. ▮▮▮ continued to have bilateral hand pain primarily in the left thumb and was seen initially at the Hand Rehabilitation Center on July 1, 1985 by Dr. ▮▮▮. Dr. ▮▮▮ diagnosed the patient as having bilateral trigger thumb, with a locked trigger thumb on the left, bilateral carpal tunnel syndrome, and degeneration of the left CMC joint of the thumb. Surgery was performed on 1/24/85 by Dr. ▮▮▮. Surgical procedures included: left trapezium implant, left carpal tunnel release, and left trigger thumb release. Ms. ▮▮▮ was seen initially in therapy at the Hand Rehabilitation Center in 2/86. At this time, she continues in both Primary Care and Work Therapy to improve the range of motion, strength and decrease pain in the left hand.

Ms. ▮▮▮ indicates that she is divorced with 4 children. She indicates that she is independent in self-care activities, but is unable to do heavy housework, lift packages, driving for long distances due to hand cramping. Her leisures activities include: gardening, sewing, and making jewelry, but the patient has not been able to perform these activities since her surgery. Ms. ▮▮▮ indicates her major difficulties are: pain and weakness in both hands, indicates the left greater than the right, and decreased ability to perform house-hold and cooking duties, such as chopping.

She reports additional medical history including: diabetes, hypertension, hiatal hernia, status post right mastectomy, chronic left ankle problem, back pain, and asthma. The patient stated she is taking insulin, Diazide, Tagamet prn, and calcium for the above conditions.

JOB HISTORY:

Ms. ▮▮▮ was employed as a nurse's aide for three years at the ▮▮▮. The Dictionary of Occupational Titles defines this job as a medium level job requiring maximum lifting of 50 lbs., with frequent lifting of 25 lbs. The physical demands of the job also include stooping, kneeling, crouching, and/or crawling, reaching, handling, fingering and/or feeling, talking and hearing, and seeing. The work environment is indoors and the employee is exposed to situations in which there is definite risk of bodily injury and possible exposure to fumes, odors, toxic conditions, dust and poor ventilation. Ms. ▮▮▮ describes the job requirements of her position as a nurse's aide as: frequently lifting patients, lifting and carrying of food trays, assisting patients with self-care, evaluating vital signs, and note-writing. Ms. ▮▮▮ reported additional job history included 6 weeks employment as a medical assistant. The patient is a high school graduate and has received certification in medical office management. Dr. Jaeger ordered the Physical Capacity Evaluation to determine Ms. ▮▮▮ physical capabilities and limitations.

The Physical Capacity Evaluation consists of three components: a Hand Function Evaluation, Administration of Standardized Tests, and Observation of Performance of Physical Demands and Job Simulation.

HAND FUNCTION EVALUATION:

Grip strength taken on the Jamar Dynamometer were as follows:

JAMAR	RIGHT HAND	LEFT HAND
Level I (tight grasp)	15 lbs.	3 lbs.
Level II	20 lbs.	13 lbs.
Level III	25 lbs.	13 lbs.
Level IV	25 lbs.	10 lbs.
Level V (wide grasp)	24 lbs.	10 lbs.

Pinch measurements were recorded with the pinch gauge. Pinch measurements were as follows:

	RIGHT HAND	LEFT HAND
Lateral Pinch:	7 lbs.	4 lbs.
Three-Point Pinch:	7 lbs.	3 lbs.

The patient experienced pain with grip and pinch testing.

PAGE THREE
RE: ████

Active range of motion measurements were recorded with the goniometer and are as follows: the right upper extremity active range of motion was within normal limits with the exception of internal rotation which was 75°, wrist extension/flexion was 60/45°. Left upper extremity active range of motion was limited at the shoulder, wrist, and hand with the following results: shoulder flexion 105° (patient reported pain with this motion), shoulder abduction 120°, internal rotation 70°, wrist extension/flexion 40/35°. The patient had full but tight thumb opposition in the left hand and she tends to substitute thumb flexion to reach the V digit. Volumetric measurements taken before and after the Physical Capacity Evaluation demonstrated that there was not a significant increase in hand volume. There actually was a 10 ml. decrease in the right hand volume and a 5 ml. increase in left hand volume. The patient was seen for the initial two-hour component of this evaluation on 5/30/86 and the evaluation was then completed on 6/10/86 due to her difficulty getting to the Hand Rehabilitation Center.

ADMINISTRATION OF STANDARDIZED TESTS:

The Valpar Upper Extremity Range of Motion Work Sample was utilized to assess the reaching, handling, and manipulating ability of each hand. Tests were performed in a confined space with vision occluded and with each hand at various positions. Ms. ████ scored in the less than 5th percentile using the Valpar San Diego Worker Norms for the dominant right hand. When working on the top panel of this Work Sample, Ms. Khoudary complained of pain in the right shoulder and elbow. After completion of the entire panel, she complained of fatigue at the base of the thumb, elbow and the shoulder. Ms. ████ was not able to complete the assembly section of this work sample with the left hand. She was unable to complete the top panel using her left hand due to left thumb and shoulder pain and therefore, the test was stopped at this time. The score of her right hand is obviously a below average score as Employed Worker Norms range from 0 to 100%.

The Valpar Whole Body Range of Motion Work Sample was used to assess the patient's ability to handle and manipulate objects while working in various body positions including bending, kneeling, and stooping with vision occluded. Ms. ████ complained of severe pain in both shoulders overhead position. The first transfer of the templates is from shoulder to waist level and she again reported severe pain in her shoulder, the left rating her pain 10 out of 10. The second transfer is from overhead to greater than the right. The third transfer requires stooping and placement of the objects in position with vision occluded. The patient was unable to complete this transfer due to severe pain in both knees.

PAGE FOUR
RE: ████

The patient was unable to complete the remainder of this test and therefore, it was discontinued at this time.

The Valpar Simulated Assembly Work Sample assesses the patient's ability to work at an assembly task requiring physical manipulation, as well as bilateral hand usage. Ms. ████ scored in the 70th percentile based upon the Valpar Method Timed Motion Standards. This score is a below average score in that Method Timed Motion Standards range from 0 to 150%.

Coordination and dexterity were assessed using the Jebson Hand Function Test. This test measures the patient's ability to write, eat, manipulate small lightweight objects, as well as circumferential 1-lb. objects. Ms. ████ scored within normal limits on placing small objects and stacking with the right hand. She scored within normal limits with the left hand in stacking tests. However, Ms. ████ scored below normal limits in writing, simulated eating, lifting, and placing objects of 1-lb. onto the test boards with both hands.

OBSERVATION OF PERFORMANCE OF PHYSICAL DEMANDS OF WORK:

Physical Task	Observation
1. Bilateral lifting	The patient was able to lift 10 lbs. maximum from floor to waist level using both hands. She reported pain in the left wrist and the shoulders bilaterally. Due to the results of the lifting evaluation from floor to waist level, additional lifting analysis was not performed. She only tolerated approximatey 2 minutes of repetitive lifting.
2. Unilateral lifting	Ms. ████ was able to lift and carry 10 lbs. maximum with the right arm a distance of 25 ft. She was unable to carry 5 lbs. unilaterally with the left hand, a distance of 25 ft., due to severe pain.
3. Pushing/pulling	The patient was not able to complete evaluation of pushing/pulling using a box at waist height. However, the patient's pushing/pulling ability was evaluated using the work simulator.
4. Reaching	The patient experienced difficulty in reaching above shoulder level, and reaching to floor level. She was able to reach at waist to shoulder level without difficulty.

5. Strength and endurance

The Work Simulator was used to evaluate static force (strength) and dynamic force (endurance) using the tool that simulates pushing/pulling. The right hand demonstrated 29% greater strength than the left hand in this test. The right hand demonstrated 7% greater average force output in the endurance testing than the left hand using the tool. However, she was unable to complete the entire test period using the right hand. On the tool that simulates repetitive gripping, the right hand demonstrated 7% greater strength than the left hand. On endurance testing using the repetitive gripping tool, the patient was unable to exert any average force output using the left hand, and was unable to complete the entire test period. The patient was able to exert light force in repetitive gripping using the right hand, but reported significant pain on the dorsal aspect of the right hand and forearm post completion of this test.

6. Grasping/handling

The results of this evaluation reveal that Ms. ▮ can use her right hand for grasping and handling of small, and light objects without significant difficulties. She can utilize her left hand for grasping small and light objects with some noted difficulty. It is significant to note that she has difficulty grasping and handling objects of medium to heavy weight with both upper extremities.

7. Manipulation

Fine manipulation is below normal limits with the right and left hands. Speed of manipulation was calculated based on the results of the Valpar Work Samples and the Jebson Hand Test utilized in this evaluation.

8. Standing, sitting, walking

Standing, sitting, and walking tolerance appeared to be slightly reduced during this two-part four-hour evaluation. There was need for several rests during this evaluation and patient reported significant fatigue and discomfort following both sections of this evaluation.

9. Climbing stairs

Ms. ▮ was able to climb 12 stairs without difficulty although she used a railing for stabilization.

10. Kneeling, crouching, crawling, stooping

Ms. ▮ was able to kneel, crouch, crawl and stoop with difficulty due to pain reported in the knees bilaterally and in the wrists.

RECOMMENDATIONS:

The patient was unable to tolerate this two-part four-hour evaluation and reported severe pain consistently in her hands, shoulders, and knees. This pain persisted for approximately 12 hours following the evaluation. The following problems were identified in this evaluation:

1. Significant pain reported consistently with any repetitive use of the hands,

2. Decreased strength in the hands bilaterally,

3. Decreased rang eof motion particularly in the left proximal upper extremity,

4. Inability to work in an overhead, stooped, or crouched position for any sustained period of time,

5. Decreased dexterity bilaterally,

6. Decreased ability to perform sedentary level lifting requirements (10 lbs.).

7. Difficulty grasping and handling of objects with the hands, left greater than right.

This evaluation was designed to evaluate the patient's ability to perform sedentary work and it is apparent that she had significant difficulty completing even two hours of sedentary level work. Therefore, it is recommended that the patient apply for Social Security Disability at this time. This is not to say, however, that the patient may be able to tolerate sedentary level work at some point in the future. However, it is strongly recommended that the work not be of the nature that involves any significant lifting of even up to 10 lbs., and any repetitive use of the hands.

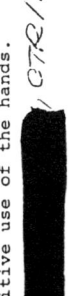

DB:ML

HAND REHABILITATION CENTER, LTD.

901 WALNUT STREET

PHILA, PA 19107

Telephone (215) 629-0980

Surgery:
James M Hunter, M.D.
Lawrence H Schneider, M.D.
Scott H Jaeger, M.D.
Stephen L Cash, M.D.

Administrator of Rehabilitation
Evelyn J. Mackin, L.P.T.

Controller
Bruce P. Cox, CPA

Hand Therapy Staff:
Barbara Goodwyn Stanley, R.P.T.
Patricia L Baxter, OTR/L
Anne D Callahan, M.S., OTR/L
Richard Bead, R.P.T.
Paula Brenne Kader, R.P.T.
Susan Toth, OTR/L
Patricia M Byron, M.A., OTR/L
Laura A Boureng, OTR/L
Susan Trihun, OTR/L
Marianne Koehler, OTR/L
Karen M Sewart, M.S., OTR/L
Gwendolyn van Stren, R.P.T.
Frank Angiolillo, R.P.T.
Gisele Larose, OTR/L
Susan Blackmore, OTR/L
Barbara L Reeder, OTR/L
Debra Beaulieu, OTR/L

PHYSICAL CAPACITY EVALUATION

NAME:

CHART: #34085-1

DATE: 5/28/86

EVALUATOR: ████████, OTR/L

HISTORY AND IDENTIFYING INFORMATION:

This 29 year-old left hand dominant male is employed as an habilitation plan coordinator and is a trained physical education instructor for New Jersey State. He has had a syndactyly of his right hand for which he has had 7-8 procedures done throughout his childhood. He states he was not followed in therapy following any of these surgical procedures.

Mr. ████ indicates that he is married, with one child. He indicates independence in all self-care areas and home care areas. He does state he will occasionally switch to his left hand for tasks he is unable to perform with his right hand. Leisure activities include all sports and coaching. He states his hand does not limit him in the performance of these things.

Mr. ████ indicates his major difficulties at present include hammering a nail, dexterity with his right hand, and manual yard work. A concern of his is for improving the cosmesis in his right hand, and his ability to gain control over little abduction and adduction. Additional medical history is significant for right wrist fracture when patient was 15 years old, right shoulder injury, and occasional back problems, as per patient report. Patient states he is taking no medications at present.

JOB HISTORY:

Mr. ████ has been employed as a physical education teacher for approximately 5 years and is now subsequently employed as an habilitation plan coordinator. He states quite a bit of his job involves public relations presently. He states there is no manual work involved but includes primarily: writing, traveling, and arranging meetings.

He states the work environment includes both inside and outside work.

The purpose of this evaluation is to determine Mr. ████ functional use of his right non dominant hand so as to appropriately discuss surgical intervention in the future.

The Physical Capacity Evaluation consists of three components: a Hand Function Evaluation, Administration of Standardized Tests, and Observation of Performance of Physical Demands.

HAND FUNCTION EVALUATION:

Grip strength measurements taken on the Jamar Dynamometer were as follows:

JAMAR	RIGHT HAND	LEFT HAND
Level I (tight grip)	25 lbs.	85 lbs.
Level II	45 lbs.	120 lbs.
Level III	48 lbs.	125 lbs.
Level IV	45 lbs.	110 lbs.
Level V (wide grip)	38 lbs.	95 lbs.

Pinch measurements recorded with the pinch meter were as follows:

	RIGHT HAND	LEFT HAND
Lateral Pinch	19 lbs.	19 lbs.
Three-Point Pinch	9 lbs.	19 lbs.
Tip Pinch:		
thumb/index	13 lbs.	15 lbs.
thumb/long	3 lbs.	15 lbs.
thumb/ring	4 lbs.	7 lbs.
thumb/little	5 lbs.	5 lbs.

COMMENTS: It should be noted that patient tends to use his right index finger quite a bit of the time and this causes occasional soreness.

Active range of motion measurements were recorded with the goniometer and are as follows:

MOTION	RIGHT HAND
Wrist ext/flex	76/65°
Rd/ud	30°/15°
thumb MP ext/flex	0/40°
IP ext/flex	0/80°
CMC abd.	35°
CMC ext.	35°
OPP	to all digits and base of V metacarpal

II   MP=   0/70°
     PIP   0/95°
     DIP   -10/50°

III MP   0/50°
     PIP   -60/100°
     DIP   no motion noted

IV   MP   0/50°
     PIP   -75/90°
     DIP   -20/30° (no active extension noted).

V   MP   0/25°
     PIP   35/100°
     DIP   -10/30°

Flex to DPC (II-V)   -3.5, -2.5, -3.5, -1.5 cm.

COMMENTS: It should be noted that he is unable to adduct his little finger and long finger extensors appear very weak.

Volumetric measurements taken before and after the evaluation demonstrated that there was not a significant increase in hand volume. This indicates that this patient tolerated three hours of manual work without swelling occurring in his hand.

ADMINISTRATION OF STANDARDIZED TESTS:

The Jebsen Hand Function Test was performed to measure coordination and dexterity. This test measures the patient's ability to write, eat, manipulate small lightweight objects, as well as circumferential 1 lb. objects with each hand. Mr. ▮▮▮ scored within norms on all 7 of the subtests for both his right and left hands. This indicates normal functional ability for activity of daily living skills. It should be noted that in prehension tasks he uses essentially a lateral pinch and for strength requirements, he uses palmar pinch. He also compensates with shoulder movement when attempting to reach some objects on the tabletop.

The Valpar Upper Extremity Range of Motion Work Sample was used to assess the reaching, handling, and manipulating ability of each hand. On 2 subtests, the right hand showed 21-39% less speed, as compared to the left hand. In the disassembly subtest, he scored below average with a 5% score, as compared to the San Diego Employed Workers Norms, between 0-100%.

Observation of his performance on this test showed him using lateral pinch with significant thumb IP flexion.

He did not favor his right hand with the disassembly task which requires both hand usage.

The Valpar Simulated Work Sample assesses a patient's ability to work at assembly tasks requiring physical manipulation, as well as bi-lateral hand usage. Normative information was not obtained on this test; however, observation of coordination was made and he did not favor his right hand as he performed the tasks equally with his right and left hands.

The Purdue Pegboard Test was utilized to measure fingertip dexterity. He scored below the 1 percentile, for right hand only, both hands, and assembly tasks. He scored within the 5th percentile for the left hand only, as compared to applicants for general factory work.

This indicates his speed for manipulation, is slow, however, he was able to manipulate the 1/8 in. objects without much effort.

OBSERVATION OF PERFORMANCE OF PHYSICAL DEMANDS OF WORK:

Physical Task	Observation
1. Lifting/carrying bilateral	1. The patient was able to lift 85 lbs. from floor to waist level using both hands.
	2. Patient was able to lift 30 lbs. from shoulder to overhead level using both hands.
	3. Patient was able to lift 30 lbs. from floor to overhead using both hands.
2. Unilateral lifting	Patient was able to lift with each hand 65 lbs. and carry for 25 ft. It should be noted that he had full grasp around both bucket handle and box with his injured right hand.
3. Pushing/pulling	Mr. ▮▮▮ was able to pull 25 lbs. with the right arm using a wall pulley for 21 repetitions, and 25 lbs. at 36 repetitions, using his left hand. He could push and pull repetitively an 85 lb. box at waist height for 3 minutes, with his right arm and additionally the same amount of weight for 3 minutes with his left hand. It should be noted the patient stated his right ring finger volar surface of his MP became somewhat sore with this task.

113

4. Reaching

Patient was able to reach in all planes of motion without difficulty.

5. Strength and Endurance

The work simulator was used to evaluate static force (strength) and dynamic force (endurance) for strength measurements. In static gripping, his right hand showed 57% less power as compared to his left hand. For a tool that simluated the use of a rake, his right hand showed 11% less static power, as compared to his left hand.

For repetitive gripping, his right hand showed 66% less power as compared to his left hand. With the tool that simulates repetitive pushing of his right hand showed 30% greater power, as compared to his left hand.

Patient described general fatigue in both extremities following this test with right fatigue greater than left.

6. Grasping/handling

Mr. ▉▉▉ can use his right hand for handling of objects which are all sizes and both light and heavy weight. His prehension pattern is noted to be essentially one of functional lateral pinch. He has no difficulty in grasping and handling any sized objects with his left hand.

7. Manipulation

Fine manipulation was below normal limits for both right and left hands as measured by the Purdue pegboard. Functional observance of this showed patient was able to perform the test, however, did perform it slowly with both hands.

8. Standing, sitting, walking

Observations of standing tolerance as estimated by the patient is thought to be 8 hours with weight shifts.

Walking tolerance is estimated to be about 3 miles. Patient also states he can jog 3 miles. Sitting tolerance is estimated to be 8-10 hours. There was no abnormal posture or gait noted. He does state that on occasion his right side becomes somewhat sore, as he feels he is overcompensating with his left for quite a few strength activities and thus causes a rotation movement in his trunk.

9. Climbing stairs/ladder

Mr. ▉▉▉ is able to climb 10 stairs 4 times without difficulty. He is able to climb a 10 ft. ladder without difficulty, 3 times. It was noted that he was able to fully support his weight with both hands on the ladder rungs.

10. Kneeling, crouching, crawling, stooping

Mr. ▉▉▉ was able to complete these tasks without difficulty. He does state that his right wrist becomes sore with repetitive push-ups.

RECOMMENDATION:

Based on Mr. ▉▉▉'s test responses, it is felt that at present he has good functional use of his hand. He is able to perform medium work as measured by his lifting tasks and use of the work simulator.

We discussed Mr. ▉▉▉ needs and desires at length on this date. His goals for any intervention include: obtaining a wider palmar area, decreasing ulnar deviation of V digit, maintaining at least his present function of his right hand, and general improvement of cosmesis, which appears to be necessary for his present job.

His strengths are his coordination abilities, which involves essentially most functional lateral pinch for this patient, as well as his strength in his right hand, which is essentially at 60% less strength as compared to his left hand. This does allow him quite a bit of functional use, however.

On this date, he was provided with several options to consider which will be discussed with his surgeon on his next doctor's visit. One of these options was a Pillet prosthesis which he could don when he needed to make public appearances. In a pre-evaluation for this prosthesis, it was felt that the flexion contractures of his ring and little finger at present might be prohibitive of the ability to don this. Thus, if this is an option to be considered, he will require intervention to increase passive extension.

We also reviewed that any surgical intervention suggested would be discussed with him upon his next doctor's appointment.

The patient does truly desire his hand to become more cosmetic, as well as maintaining good function.

SB:ML

Reprinted with permission from the Hand Rehabilitation Center, Ltd., Philadelphia, PA.

HAND REHABILITATION CENTER, LTD.

901 WALNUT STREET
PHILA, PA 19107

Telephone (215) 629-0980

Surgery:
James M. Hunter, M.D.
Lawrence H. Schneider, M.D.
Scott H. Jaeger, M.D.
Stephen L. Cash, M.D.

Administrator of Rehabilitation
Evelyn J. Mackin, L.P.T.

Hand Therapy Staff:
Paula Breme Kader, R.P.T.
Patricia Baxter Petralia, M.S., O.T.R./L.
Anne D. Callahan, M.S., O.T.R./L.
Susan Toth, R.P.T./L.
Richard Reed, R.P.T.
Patricia M. Byron, M.A., O.T.R./L.
Laura A. Bruening, O.T.R./L.
Marianne Koehler, O.T.R./L.
Karen M. Stewart, M.S., O.T.R./L.
Gwendolyn van Strien, R.P.T.
Frank Angiolillo, R.P.T.
Gisele Larose, O.T.R./L.
Susan Blackmore, M.S., O.T.R./L.
Colleen Burke, P.T.A.
Jane Mangiarelli, P.T.

TO:

FROM: Hand Rehabilitation Center
901 Walnut Street
Philadelphia, PA 19107

RE: ON-SITE JOB ASSESSMENT

An on-site job assessment was performed at ████████ on February 18 1987. Observation of various assembly line tasks and automated packing machine tasks were made as identified below. The primary focus was identification of the most appropriate jobs that an employee could perform if he or she had a history of carpal tunnel syndrome. Recommendations were also made for prevention of carpal tunnel and other problems by reducing repetitive motion, encouraging proper work positions and reinforcing good work habits.

I. Red Case Packing Stock

A. OBSERVATIONS

1. Lifting cardboard sheets and stacking sheets into boxes using wrist flexion (bending of wrist down), ulnar deviation, (wrist movement toward little finger) and repetitive static pinching with thumb index and long finger.

2. Pressure to the base of the palms when placing lids on boxes.

3. Lifting and turning 180° to place 10 lb. candy box on the rack.

RECOMMENDATIONS:

1. Place loops on the cardboard to prevent unwanted wrist motions and to prevent static pinching of the thumb, index and long fingers.

Employee would slide hand through the loops using the desired wrist position and avoiding the pinching of the fingers.

2. Replace currently used cardboard sheets with a sturdier cardboard sheet which can be grasped with less force while pinching and lifting.

3. Instruct employees to not bang their palms on lids that do not fit on easily.

4. Instruct employees to place lid on using ulnar (little finger side of hand) aspect of hands with the wrist in a neutral position. See diagram below.

5. Wear mits which have a gel pad insert in the palm to distribute pressure when placing lids on boxes. See picture attached.

6. Have employees always lift 10 lb. red case boxes with two hands to prevent excessive loading to one group of arm muscles.

7. Place racks on the down side of conveyor belt next to the employee, so that employee will only be required to do a half turn thereby, reducing length of time he/she is carrying a 10 lb. red case.

*Note: This is a very heavy, repetitive job, that would not be ideal for an employee with a history of carpal tunnel syndrome.

8. Each employee stamps tags approximately 1,200 times daily. This supplies a repetitive hard impact to the palm. An automatic stamper or varied color cards could reduce this stress.

II. Straight Line Belt

A. OBSERVATIONS

1. Employees remove lids from the white boxes two at a time with wrists bent in the flexed and ulnar deviated position.

2. The paper cups do not always separate easily, so employees must use repetitive static pinching of thumb, index and long fingers.

3. When placing candy pieces into the box on the conveyor belt, the employee must reach an excessive distance due to the counter space in front of the conveyor belt.

4. The cartoner worker was noted to be lifting several boxes at a time.

115

Dear Colleague:

This year I have had the opportunity to work at an industrial site as a consultant in the Human Factors Program. The Human Factors Program consists of the coordinated efforts of an ergonomics engineer, the medical doctor in charge of evaluation and treatment of the employees, a physical therapist consultant, and occupational therapy consultant, and the nursing staff of the company. We have worked together developing and modifying several factors to this program.

The program is called a Human Factors Program because each employee's physical performance and adjustment to his work is analyzed based on his own individual response. The work sites for each employee are modified according to the needs of the person. An example of this is if the short person sits in a chair and he cannot touch the floor comfortably with his feet, he will tend to experience fatigue in his lower extremities. A simple work site modification is provision of a footstool to prevent this fatigue. Most of these modifications are designed by the ergonomics engineer. The occupational therapist gives input to the engineer on the medical problems which can occur from the posture the employees have developed.

Other parts of this program which were very helpful to the employees include:

1. Exercise program for all employees provided ten minutes, three times a day during the work schedule. This program alleviates fatigue, prevents tenosyno-vitis, and increases flexibility and strength. The exercises consist of active stretching exercises, isotonic strengthening exercises and isometric strengthening exercises.

2. In addition to the daily exercise program on the floor, employees are provided with daily therapy if a physical problem has developed. The majority of these treated have cumulative trauma disorders due to the repetitive nature of their work. All types of modalities are utilized to provide therapy which is effective for each individual. The employees are provided with static splints for rest of an inflamed part or to support a part during functional use. Therapy also includes strengthening exercises and exercises to alleviate swelling and compression of the peripheral nerves.

Consulting in an industrial setting is a great learning experience for the therapist. It is an experience that moves the therapist into the realm of facilitating functional use and maintaining the employee in his work environment. It has been beneficial for the therapist and the employees.

Patricia Baxter, O.T.R./L.

PB:me

B. RECOMMENDATIONS:

1. Instruct employees to remove lids one at a time and to lift the lids off from the side of the box. If done correctly this would not decrease production time. Reducing the undesired wrist motion.

2. Have employees wear finger cots while separating cups; this will reduce frictional force on the thumb, index and long fingers.

3. Have a "U" cut out in counter so that employees can sit closer to the conveyor belt. This will enable employees to work with hands and arms in the proper work position. Place the candy either to the left or to the right of the employee.

4. Lifting several boxes at one time is faster for the cartoner. However, both hands should be used. This will reduce stress on the hands and wrists and should not decrease productivity.

*Note: Employees who have a history of carpal tunnel syndrome could wear custom made support splints which will prevent them from bending their wrist into undesirable positions.

The padder, lidder, wrapper and band wrapper are all tasks that an employee with a history of carpal tunnel syndrome/release could possibly perform. We would recommend that the employee wear a custom made support splint which we have prescribed previously.

III. Automatic Packing Machine

A. OBSERVATION:

1. The automatic packing machine operator was observed lifting the red case boxes with one arm.

2. One employee was observed manually placing candies in boxes. She did this without adapting any stressful wrist or hand positions and her work was placed at an appropriate distance from her.

B. RECOMMENDATIONS:

1. Instruct employees to carry the 10 lb. red case with two hands reducing static loading on one group of muscles.

2. The manual placement of candies (following automatic packing of other candies) is a possible job for a worker with carpal tunnel syndrome/release history.

116

ON-SITE JOB ANALYSIS

GENERAL INFORMATION: This thirty-five year old packer for ▓▓▓▓▓▓▓▓ Products Corporation reportedly developed gradual onset of symptoms of numbness and tingling in both arms starting in March, 1990. She had EMG findings which were positive for carpal tunnel syndrome bilaterally. The patient underwent right carpal tunnel release on 11/5/90 and left carpal tunnel release on 12/11/90. At the time of the initial evaluation at the Northeast Work Hardening Center on 6/13/91, the patient reported complaints of numbness and weakness of her right and left arm. She complained of frequently dropping items and muscle twitching with both arms. The patient has participated in therapy for the past five weeks and presently is performing a strengthening program to improve her posture and endurance of both arms. On 7/17/91, ▓▓▓▓▓▓ had requested an on-site job analysis to be performed to determine whether the patient could perform at her regular job or a modified job at ▓▓▓▓▓ Products Corporation.

CLINICAL PICTURE

Functional Status: The patient's cervical active range of motion measured 70 deg. cervical rotation to the right and 75 deg. to the left. Lateral flexion measured 45 deg. to the right and 55 deg. to the left. The patient lacked 1-1/4" touching her sternum notch with her chin during cervical flexion. Active range of motion of her right wrist measured: flexion 60 deg., extension 62 deg., radial deviation 25 deg., ulnar deviation 30 deg., supination 65 deg., and pronation 90 deg. Active range of motion of the left wrist measured: flexion 60 deg., extension 70 deg., radial deviation 35 deg., ulnar deviation 35 deg., supination 68 deg. and pronation 90 deg. Grip strength measured 44 lbs in the right hand and 35 lbs in the left hand. Lateral pinch measured 17 lbs right thumb and 17 lbs bilaterally. Three point pinch measured 14 lbs right hand and 15 lbs left hand. ▓▓▓▓ is using a clavical strap to assist in retracting her shoulders and improving her posture.

Limitations: The patient reports she will have difficulty pulling the parts out of the Gaylord to pack them. Job simulation has not been incorporated in the patient's therapy program as of yet. Further limitations will be defined in the therapy progress notes.

PHYSICAL PLANT

Hours of Operation: The plant has three eight-hour shifts. There are two ten-minute breaks and one fifteen-minute paid lunch break.

Physical Demands of Jobs Available:

▓▓▓▓▓▓, the Plant Supervisor of ▓▓▓▓▓▓ Products Corporation, explained the physical demands of five jobs available to Karen in the plant. These jobs include:

1. Packer: The physical demands of packer requires the person to stand or sit while pulling metal parts from Gaylords and stacking them in specific orders to arrange them in cardboard boxes. The metal pieces can weight from one to six ounces. A rod is available to pull the pieces out of the Gaylord. The rod is approximately 3 ft. long. Some of the metal parts are tangled and difficult to sort. The packer pulls out the pieces, counts them, nests them and puts them in a carton. The carton is made up by the packer. An average of 20 cartons are assembled per hour. The boxes are stacked from waist height onto a Gaylord. The boxes can range in size from 6 X 7 X 2-3/4" to 21" X 11" X 10". The weight of the boxes range from 2 oz. to 35 lbs.

ON-SITE JOB EVALUATION

Re:
WC:

On August 8, 1988, an on-site job evaluation was performed for ▓▓▓▓▓. The contact person was ▓▓▓▓▓▓▓▓, the night operation manager. The job title of relief operator. The length of the shift is 8 hours.

The physical demands of the job are as follows: lifting minimal weight of 5 lbs. at a frequency of 400 times per day. Maximal weight to be lifted is 80 lbs. with a frequency of 400 per day. The average weight lifted is 50 lbs. with a frequency of 27,000 times per day.

Lifting range: minimal weight from waist level to above head. Maximal weight from waist level to waist level. Average weight from floor to above head.

Objects Lifted: milk crates, half-gallon containers and boxes.

Carrying: minimal 10 lbs. with a frequency of 3 times per day a distance of 10 feet. Maximally 80 lbs. with a frequency of 400 times with a distance of 10 feet.

Reaching: frequently overhead activity is performed 400 to 27,000 times per day.

Pulling: minimal weight of 300 lbs. 60 times per day.

Tools Used: wrench on the average of 2 times per day for 10 minute periods.

Depending on the job to be performed by ▓▓▓, standing and sitting activities varied from 50% to 100% during the day. Climbing ladders were also part of job performance, the ladder was 8 feet high with side rails.

The job environment was indoors and outdoors.

This job evaluation permitted us to determine that 4 out of the 5 jobs observed required overhead reaching. The only job that did not require this was the Fedroll.

Reprinted with permission
from the Hand Rehabilitation
Center, Ltd. of Philadelphia
PA

117

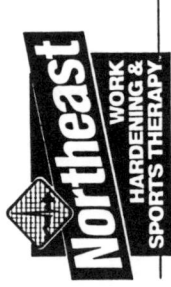

Northeast WORK HARDENING & SPORTS THERAPY

July 12, 1991

Dear ____:

On July 11, 1991, measurements were taken to determine the forces required to operate an ____ splicing machine. Listed below are the job tasks analyzed and the forces measured for operation:

JOB TASK	FORCES
1. wire insertion in modules	5.65 lbs.
2. lever operation	43.67 lbs.

Please note, that the above forces were obtained using a Isometric Work Analyzer. If you have any questions, please do not hesitate to call on us. We look forward to working with you in the future.

PB:wam

2. **Assembly of Elbows:** Elbows made of copper or metal weight up to 1 lbs. Elbows are dumped from a Gaylord to a tilt table. The full Gaylords weight between 35 and 50 lbs. Three hundred to four hundred elbows are packed into boxes each hour. This position also requires cutting of elbows. The crank of the saw is turned at shoulder level with the right arm. The vise can be pushed with the hip and tightened with the left hand. The operator must stack, push and pull Gaylords which are used to store elbows.

3. **Fabricating Samples:** The employee is required to clean the samples, sand to free them from burrs, place the siding on one side of the bifold and the color chips on the other side. Adhesive is applied to the 3' by 5' board to assemble chips in a display. The boards vary in dimension from 4' X 4' to 2' X 2'. A drill is used to assemble the parts on the display board. A saw is used to run long pieces of siding through to cut to specified dimensions. The employee is required to feed the pieces onto the ripped fence of the saw. This job requires alternating between sawing, deburring and using the paper cutter.

4. **Grinding** The employee is required to push pieces of siding into a grinding machine repetitively. The siding is stacked on a pallet. Also, sweeping to clean the area is required once a day.

5. **Packing Siding:** The employee is required to stand and pick up two pieces of siding at a time, flip them over and then lift and push them into a cardboard box. Twenty pieces of siding are packed into each box. The boxes weigh 80 lbs when they are full of siding. Packing of the boxes is required from knee level to shoulder level height. The employee is required to pull the wheel chuck out and pull the cart out or push it with her foot. Ends are placed on the cardboard boxes and secured with a compressed air staple gun. Wrist flexion combined with forearm supination and pronation is required to position the staple gun correctly to operate it. The operator is required to pick up trash and sweep the area to clean it. The employee also inspects each piece of siding as it is lifted into the boxes. Hand motions required in this job include intrinsic plus position, pistol grip and palmar grip.

RECOMMENDATIONS:

The job demands of the five available jobs will be simulated in therapy to determine the patient's physical ability and endurance to perform each one. A follow-up report will be provided on the patient's physical abilities and restrictions.

PB:mw

cc: ____ Products Corp.

118

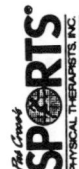

HAND REHABILITATION CENTER. LTD.
901 WALNUT STREET
PHILADELPHIA, PA 19107
Telephone (215) 629-0980

Surgery
James M. Hunter, M.D.
Lawrence H. Schneider, M.D.
Stephen L. Gab, M.D.
Daniel J. Singer, M.D.

Administrator of Rehabilitation
Evelyn J. Mackin, L.PT.

Hand Therapy
Patricia Baxt...
Paula Breme
Richard Read
Patricia M. B
Laura A. Bru
Frank Angiolino, R.PT.
Susan Blackmore, M.S., OTR.L
Colleen Burke, PT.A.
Jane Mangarelli, PT
Patricia A. Wright, MOT. OTR.L
Julie Belkin, OTR.L.CO

October 29, 1987

RE: ▇▇▇▇▇▇▇▇▇

Dear Mr. ▇▇▇▇▇▇▇▇▇:

Enclosed you will find the Physical Capacity Evaluation on your client ▇▇▇▇▇▇▇. If you have any questions, please don't hesitate to contact me.

Sincerely,

Patricia Baxter, OTR/L

Patricia Baxter, OTR/L

PB:lh
Enclosure

HAND REHABILITATION CENTER. LTD.
901 WALNUT STREET
PHILADELPHIA, PA 19107
Telephone (215) 629-0980

M.D.

Administrator of Rehabilitation:
Evelyn J. Mackin, L.PT.

Hand Therapy Staff:
Patricia Baxter Petralia, M.S. OTR./L
Paula Breme Kadir, R.PT
Richard Read, R.PT
Patricia M. Byron, M.A., OTR./L
Laura A. Bruening, OTR./L.
Frank Angiolillo, R.PT.
Susan Blackmore, M.S., OTR. L
Colleen Burke, PT.A
Jane Mangarelli, PT
Patricia A. Wright, MOT. OTR.L
Julie Belkin, OTR.L.CO

PHYSICAL CAPACITY EVALUATION

NAME: ▇▇▇▇▇▇▇▇▇

CHART#: 35010-8

DATE: OCTOBER 13, 1987

EVALUATOR: PATRICIA BAXTER, M.S., OTR/L

MEDICAL HISTORY AND IDENTIFYING INFORMATION:

This 28 year old, right hand dominant male was employed at Five Star Linen on August 21, 1986 when he sustained a crush injury to his right upper extremity in a machine. Surgery was performed and included:

1. 8-21-86 - Right forearm fasciotomy

2. 8-26-86 - Debridement and skin graft to right forearm.

3. 9-2-86 - Debridement and skin grafting right forearm.

4. 6-9-87 - Capsulotomy right thumb carpometacarpal joint.

Mr. ▇▇▇▇▇▇▇ was followed in therapy at the Hand Rehabilitation Center from September 3, 1986 to the present time. He presently performs a home program of exercises and continues to attend therapy twice monthly for evaluation and instructions in a home program. He returned to work on July 24, 1987.

119

-2-

Mr. ▓ indicates he is married with no children. He indicates independence in self care and home care activities. He stated his physical limitations of the right upper extremity include: difficulty lifting heavy objects, difficulty handling tools with the right hand, difficulty repairing machines due to limited right wrist motion, and difficulty manipulating small objects such as nuts and bolts with the right hand. Mr. ▓ also reported difficulty playing tennis, golfing, and skiing since his injury. He reported he utilizes a builtup handle on the sports equipment.

Mr. ▓ states his major complaints with the right upper extremity include: lack of a tight fisted grip of the right hand, weakness of pinch of the right thumb, index finger, ring finger, long finger, and small finger, pain in the right wrist with forceful use, and fatigue in the right thumb muscles with use. He has no additional medical history which limits his functional capacity. He is presently not taking any medication.

JOB HISTORY:

Mr. ▓ was employed and continues to be employed as the manager of ▓ company. He has worked at this job for the past three years. Prior to managing this company, he had worked in a laundry.

Mr. ▓ describes the job requirements of managing a laundry as: supervising staff, loading and unloading washers with 600 lbs. of linen, pulling sheets and towels from the washers and dryers, pushing carts weighing up to 600 lbs., sorting, folding laundry, distributing chemicals in machines, writing 20 minutes a day and talking on the telephone for sales. The Dictionary of Occupational Titles defines this job as sedentary work requiring lifting of 10 pounds and includes the physical requirements of reaching, handling, manipulating, and feeling. When the manager participates in the operation of the laundry, the job physical demands also include stooping, kneeling, crouching, crawling, reaching, handling, manipulating, and feeling.

The Physical Capacity Evaluation consists of three components: a hand function evaluation, administration of standardized test, and observation of performance of physical demands and job simulation.

HAND FUNCTION EVALUATION:

Grip strength taken on the Jamar Dynamometer were as follows:

-3-

JAMAR DYNAMOMETER	RIGHT HAND	LEFT HAND
Level I(tight grip)	25 lbs.	70 lbs.
Level II	40 lbs.	112 lbs.
Level III	49 lbs.	110 lbs.
Level IV	55 lbs.	95 lbs.
Level V(wide grip)	45 lbs.	90 lbs.

Pinch measurements were recorded with the pinch meter. Pinch measurements were as follows:

Lateral Pinch	Right Hand	Left Hand
Thumb/Index	9 lbs.	24 lbs.

Tip Pinch:

	Right Hand	Left Hand
Thumb/Index	4 lbs.	12 lbs.
Thumb/Long	5 lbs.	14 lbs.
Thumb/Ring	3 lbs.	12 lbs.
Thumb/Little	Unable	9 lbs.

Active range of motion measurements were recorded with the goniometer as follows:

Right wrist flexion: 25°
Left wrist flexion: 80°

Right wrist extension: 35°
Left wrist extension: 50°

Right wrist radial deviation: 5°
Left wrist radial deviation: 15°

Right wrist ulnar deviation: 15°
Left wrist ulnar deviation: 25°

Right wrist supination: 75°
Left wrist supination: 90°

Right and left wrist pronation: 90°

Left metacarpophalangeal joints of index, middle, ring, and little measured 90, 90, 95, and 95°; right metacarpopha-langeal joints of index 65, middle 75°, ring 70°, and little 80°; left proximal interphalangeal joints measured index 95, middle 98, ring 100, and little finger 100°; right proximal interphalangeal joints measured index 85°, middle 110°, ring finger 80°, little finger 95°; left distal interphalangeal joints measured 75 index, 80 middle, 85 ring, and 70 little finger; right distal interphalangeal joints measured index 60°, middle 80°, ring 70°, and little finger 25°; left digits touched distal palmar crease of palm fully; right digits touched distal palmar crease with index and long finger and lacked 2cm with the ring finger and 2.5cm with the little finger.

120

sensibility evaluation included measurement of light touch, deep pressure, and prehension speed with vision occluded. Light touch perception normal (2.86) in the right and left hands except for loss of protective sensation in the right thumb and the right forearm at the skin graft site. Speed of prehension was 7.9 seconds with the right hand and 6.8 seconds with the left hand when Mr. ███ picked up 9 objects while looking at them and placed them in a box. With his vision blocked, speed was diminished with the right hand to 19.6 seconds and 14.9 seconds with the left hand.

Volumetric measurements taken before and after the Physical Capacity Evaluation demonstrated that there was not a significant increase in hand volume after the patient used his hands for three hours. Hand volume recorded before the patient worked measured 515ml in the right hand and 520ml in the left hand. After he completed the test, hand volume measured 525ml in the right hand and 510ml in the left hand. Normally hand volume decreases with active use.

ADMINISTRATION OF STANDARDIZED TEST:

The Valpar Whole Body Range of Motion Work Sample was used to assess the patient's ability to handle and manipulate objects while working in various body positions including bending, kneeling, and stooping with vision occluded. Mr. Guttman scored in the 95th percentile using both hands on the Valpar Work Sample and comparing his score to the Valpar San Diego Employed Worker Norms. This score is above average as compared to Employed Worker Norms which range from 0 to 100%. Mr. ███ was observed compensating by using his left hand for the majority of the work during this test. Mr. ███ complained of significant fatigue and discomfort in his right shoulder, wrist, and digits after 5 minutes of working. The test required approximately 20 minutes to complete.

The Valpar Small Tools Mechanical Work Sample measures the patient's ability to work with small tools. On the panel requiring right handed tool use, the patient scored in the 5th percentile using San Diego Employed Worker Norms. This score is a below average score as Employed Worker Norms range from 0 to 100%. On the panel requiring left handed tool use, the patient scored in the 90th percentile. This score is an above average score as Employed Worker Norms range from 0 to 100%.

Coordination and dexterity were assessed using the Jebsen Taylor Hand Function Test. This test measures that patient's ability to write, eat, manipulate small lightweight objects, as well as circumferential one pound objects.

Mr. ███ scored within normal limits on 7 of the 7 test components with his left hand. He scored below normal limits with the right hand on picking up small objects.

OBSERVATION OF PERFORMANCE OF PHYSICAL DEMANDS OF WORK:

Physical Task	Observation
1. Lifting/Carrying	Mr. ███ was able to lift and carry 91 lbs. with his left hand and the same amount of weight with his right hand a distance of 25 ft. He was able to lift and carry 107 pounds using both arms.
2. Reaching	Mr. ███ was able to reach forward, at waist level, and overhead without difficulty with his right and left arms. Endurance was good for left arm reaching and fair for right arm reaching. He was able to reach with his left arm without discomfort for 20 minutes whereas with his right arm he experienced discomfort after 5 minutes of reaching.
3. Grasping/Handling	Mr. ███ can use his right hand for grasping and handling of heavy sized objects without difficulty. He experiences difficulty when he attempts to grasp and handle small and light sized objects with his right hand. With his left hand he can grasp and handle small, light, and heavy sized objects without difficulty.
4. Manipulation	Fine manipulation with within normal limits with the left hand. Right hand manipulation was below normal limits. Difficulty with manipulation with the right hand is due to poor strength of the thumb muscles which limit opposition.

-6-

5. Standing, Sitting Walking

Standing tolerance is estimated by Mr. ▓▓▓▓▓ to be 8 hours. Walking tolerance is estimated to be 5 miles. Sitting tolerance is estimated to be 8 hours. There was normal body posture observed.

6. Climbing Stairs

Mr. ▓▓▓▓ was able to climb stairs without difficulty.

7. Kneeling, Crouching, Crawling, Stooping

Mr. ▓▓▓ was able to kneel, crouch, and stoop without difficulty. Crawling was awkward due to inability to place the right hand palm on the floor surface.

8. Endurance

Endurance was tested using the Work Simulator. It is a computerized evaluation instrument that can measure the power omitted by the hands and arms with a variety of tools. Mr. ▓▓▓▓'s right hand scored 50% less endurance than his left hand on the tool that requires repetitive gripping. On the tool that simulates repetitive screwdriver use, Mr. ▓▓▓▓ right hand demonstrated 60% less endurance than his left hand.

SUMMARY:

Based on Mr. ▓▓▓▓▓▓▓ test response, it appears he exerted his maximum effort during this 4 hour evaluation. Measurements of his hand function indicate grip strength of the right hand is 50% less than the left hand. Pinch strength is also diminished in the right hand. Pinch strength measured 1/3 strength in the right hand compared to the left hand. Range of motion is decreased in the right digits and thumb.

-7-

sensation of the right thumb and right forearm skin graft is loss of protective sensation. Coordination is diminished in the right hand compared to the left hand. Finally, endurance is diminished in the right hand compared to the left hand.

Patricia Baxter, OTR/L

PATRICIA BAXTER, OTR/L

PB:lh

PROFESSIONAL OCCUPATIONAL THERAPY SERVICES

2727 HOUMA BOULEVARD   —   TELEPHONE 504/455-7093

METAIRIE, LOUISIANA 70006

SUSAN L. SMITH, M.A., L.O.T.R., F.A.O.T.A.
DIRECTOR

BARBARA C. LEBLANC, M.ED., L.O.T.R.
STAFF

****

05/20/91

FUNCTIONAL EVALUATION

Mr. ******, a 43 year old man, had been referred for a Functional Evaluation. Upon his arrival he showed obvious sign of disability in that he was walking with a cane. He had come from his home in Lumberton, Mississippi. He was accompanied by his wife who had driven him.

Throughout the three hour evaluation Mr. ****** was fully cooperative with all that was asked of him. That despite the fact that during the performance component of this evaluation he was in extreme pain.

The Functional Evaluation consists of three components. These are as follows.

1. Review of Medical Documentation: This review is done in order for the therapist to learn of the client's pathology, any medical contra-indications there might be for activity, and medical prognosis.

2. Activity Interview: The activity interview ascertains the client's general life style level of activity and post injury level of activity. Topics covered are work history, educational background, family and home responsibilities, leisure time interests, and capabilities for personal care.

3. Performance Component: This assessment is selected depending upon what residual problems the client exhibits. As the client's condition affects his whole body functioning, the Smith Physical Capacities Evaluation was chosen for this portion. This assessment measures the way a person utilizes their body as a whole in being able to meet the physical demands of activity.

ACTIVITY INTERVIEW:

Mr. ****** states that he has a fourth grade education. At this time he states that his academic abilities are extremely limited. He can only read a very few words. He is able to write his name and address but unable to write a simple message or anything beyond this personal information. He is able to tell time and read a ruler to one half inches. He states that he is able to make personal change with "pretty good" ability. He states that at this time he is further limited in his ability to

---

FUNCTIONAL EVALUATION
Page 2

05/20/91

attempt to do anything such as read a few words or write as his vision is poor. All job skills have been learned through on the job training.

Mr. ****** states that he has had three occupations throughout his career life. At one point he was a fleet truck operator. His responsibilities for this job were to change tires for a fleet of heavy equipment. Then he states that he has worked alternately as a construction laborer and as a roughneck, both on and off shore. His most regular work in the past 10 to 12 years has been as a roughneck. The only other work experience the client has had is that when he served in the National Guard. He states that this was at a time about 15 to 16 years ago. He was assigned in the supply area during his National Guard duty.

At the time of his injury the client states that he was working as a roughneck in the offshore oil industry. He related that he has found that he has been unable to work since that time. He related concern about his future and ability to work. He states that he realizes that he perhaps can never return to heavy and active work which he has done in the past. He also stated that he is concerned that perhaps the only jobs that he may able to meet the physical demands for will be jobs performed inside. He states that he cannot tolerate working or being inside for long periods of time. He thinks he is claustrophobic.

Mr. ****** states that he is married and has three children. He has sons 12 and 13 years old and a daughter 12. His son and daughter are twins. The family live in a house with a yard and barnyard animals. Prior to his injury the client states that he took the responsibility for all the yard care. Now he finds that he cannot meet these physical demands to care for the yard. Consequently he supervises his sons. He states that they are able to minimumly care for the yard which is basically adequate.

As for the household activities of cooking, shopping, laundry, and cleaning the client states that he has always shared these responsibilities with his wife on an approximate 50/50 basis. He related that his wife has never been in good health and consequently at times she has been unable to do much of the household activities. At this time Mr. ****** states that he finds that he cannot assist in any of these activities. Consequently, in order to assist his wife, his sister-in-law shares these with his wife. His sister-in-law lives very close by.

The childcare responsibilities have always been shared by the couple. Mr. ****** states that many of the family's activities are oriented toward their children. He states that the relationship between a father and his son is of great importance. He related that this comradity relationship developed with his being able to play ball, wrestle, etc. with his children as well as engage in other activities. Now he finds that he cannot engage in these play activities with his sons. He finds this "aggravating" as well as his children find it the same. Another activity which the client related that he did with his

123

children was to take them hunting with him in order to "train" them to be able to hunt safely. He now cannot do this and his brother-in-law has taken over.

The client states that all his routine auto maintenance as well as all mechanical work on his vehicle he did himself prior to his injury. At this time he finds that he cannot do any of the maintenance nor mechanical work. He related that his oldest son is very much interested in auto mechanics and he is supervising him to do the routine maintenance. However he does not feel that he is able enough to do any of the mechanical work at this time.

The barnyard animals which the family have are a variety of yard and house dogs. They include Boston Terriers and Chihuahuas. The client states that he has taken the responsibility for bathing the Boston Terriers and Chihuahuas. He continues to be able to do this as they are well behaved and small. There are three hog pigs. He states that the two sows are ready to have piglets. The client states that he will be unable to do the necessary separation of the mother's from the babies, etc. He is depending upon his sons to do this for this event. Additionally the client has 40 guinea hens and about 25-30 laying hens. He finds that he is unable to feed the hogs but is able to feed the hens and collect the eggs. His sons ready a light plastic pail of feed for him. This weighs approximately 3-4 pounds. He is then able to scatter the feed out to the hens.

Additionally the client states that he always has had a large garden. He has found that this year he was unable to plant the garden. His sons and his mother-in-law planted a small garden. His wife and he would take the responsibility for the garden and can the produce for use during the winter. As well the client states that he has about 55 fruit trees. These include quince, peaches, pears, plums, and blueberries. These require spraying every two weeks in order to produce satisfactory fruit. The client states that this year he has been unable to want his sons to attempt it. The little fruit which will be produced this year he expects that his children, wife, and mother-in-law will pick. He finds that he cannot assist in this endeavor.

The client states that his leisure interests have always revolved around his home and family. He states that he has always enjoyed hunting, both gun and bow hunting. Neither of these is he able to do at this time. He also has enjoyed fishing from a boat. He states that he has only gone once since his injury. He has gone with his brother-in-law who has done all the work related to putting the boat in, operating it, etc. On that day the large fish were not biting. They only caught small fish and he found that he was able to handle them satisfactorily. Other than these two activities he states that he has always enjoyed playing ball and other activities with his children and doing the housework. Also he has always enjoyed working in the garden and with his animals. All of these activities have now

124

been severely restricted. Additionally the client states that each summer he would assist with Bible School and would regularly visit Parishioners who were sick once a week. He also regularly has attended Sunday services. At this time the client states that he has only been able to make one visitation since his injury. His attendance at Sunday services has been irregular due to his discomfort. As well his wife has not been well and he has stayed with her. He is uncertain if he will be able to participate in Bible School this summer. He states that his usual job is to oversee the children's behavior in classes. He states that at times, especially the teenagers, get quite restless. As this does not involve a great deal of physical activity he believes, if this is his assignment, that he may be able to continue to assist this summer.

The client has both a small pick up truck and a car. He related that he is unable to drive his truck with a standard transmission. Therefore it has been left parked since his injury. The only driving which the client does not is occasionally to a store. This is about two miles from his home. He related that he cannot maintain his right foot on the accelerator as it is too painful to his groin and the leg tends to become stiff. Also with his vision poor he does not want to risk much driving. He also states that if he maintains his gaze he tends to develop severe headaches. The car has an automatic transmission, power brakes and steering. Today Mrs. ****** drove the client to his appointment. He states that if his wife is unable to drive his mother-in-law will drive him to necessary errands and appointments.

In his personal care activities of dressing, bathing, grooming, and feeding the client states that he continues to be independent. He proceeds at a slow pace and has modified some of his means of accomplishing the activities. He states that any time when he has a headache he is incapacitated. If this should occur during a time when he is involved with personal care he states that he must lay down until it passes.

PERFORMANCE COMPONENT:

On the Physical Capacity Evaluation Mr. ****** showed himself to be extremely limited in his ability to meet the physical demands of activity. Limiting him was the development of severe pain in his right groin area which radiated to his right low back. Also his standing and walking balance is limited. In all activities tested the client had fair to poor endurance. Any activity which he has weight bearing on his right leg and/or has flexion of his right hip he tolerates poorly. This is nearly all activity. The greater the weight bearing and the greater degree of flexion of the hip the more severe the pain. It was seen that Mr. ****** can handle weights only on a very occasional basis of less than 5 pounds. He cannot handle these weights in the overhead or low planes. His functional sitting and standing tolerance is minimal. As well his non-functional standing tolerance is very limited. However he is able to sit in a non-functional position for up to 1 to 2 hours. The client's hand grasp in both hand is in the poor range.

For details of Mr. ******'s performance on the Physical Capacity Evaluation see that portion of this report.

MEDICAL DOCUMENTATION:

This therapist has for review numerous medical reports. They date from 9-2-90 through March 18, 1991. From these reports it is learned that the client suffered a fall. The diagnoses have been the following:

1. _____, M.D., 10-03-90:

   o Syncope
   o History of Closed Head Trauma
   o Cervical and Lumbar Pain

2. _____, M.D., 12-05-90:

   o Patient developed fribromyositis...with continued lumbar strain

3. _____ M.D., February 26, 1991:

   o Possible post-traumatic vascular headaches but suspected strong psychological overlay...

4. _____, M.D., 03-18-91.

   o Lumbar Disc Rupture Syndrome with Radiculopathy
   o Occipital Neuralgia

These reports indicate that Mr. ****** has been treated conservatively with physical therapy and medication.

The client, today, stated that since his injury he has developed glaucoma. Included in the reports which this therapist has for review there is no documentation relative to ophthalmology concerns. However from his description of this concern and treatment it appears that he is being followed by a physician.

OPINION:

Mr. ****** is a man in his mid mid career years. He has worked at heavy and physically active work throughout his career life. At this time he is unable to meet the physical demands of any activity beyond personal care and extremely light daily life activity. The medical reports are not specific as to a prognosis for Mr. ******. There is a recommendation for further diagnostic study. Specifically lumbar myelography is recommended by Dr. Jarrott. Therefore it appears that Mr. ****** has not reached his maximum medical benefit if diagnostic studies indicate further medical and/or surgical intervention. Conversely if they

do not show this indication then perhaps Mr. ****** has reached his maximum medical benefit. In order for him to return to any type of competitive employment he would need to dramatically improve his tolerance for activity. Mr. ****** cannot be projected to return to any type of work, even if his physical condition dramatically improved, except that which is manual in nature. That is due to his being illiterate and at an age when it is not feasible for him to upgrade his educational background to a significant level for work activity.

In summary it is seen that Mr. ****** has had numerous job opportunities available to him. These specifically manually oriented. At this time he cannot meet the physical demands for any competitive work, whether it be wholly sedentary or more active. His level of activity at this point is personal care and very light daily life activity. Unless his pain dramatically dissipates it can be projected that he will not be able to return to the competitive labor market. Concerns relative to his possible eye problems may also be a factor to consider in return to work. That is in the event that he gets to a point where his pain has dramatically dissipated. Therefore, the job opportunities which have been open to Mr. ****** in the past may now have been closed or at best severely curtailed.

125

PHYSICAL CAPACITY EVALUATION

NAME: ▮▮▮▮▮▮▮▮▮▮▮

CHART#: 367136

DATE: January 10, 1989

EVALUATOR: Patricia Baxter, MS, OTR/L

MEDICAL HISTORY AND IDENTIFYING INFORMATION:

This 21 year old, right hand dominant female student sustained a crush injury on March 20, 1986 to her right III and IV fingertips resulting in laceration and fractures. The patient's fingertips were crushed in a shopping cart accident in the parking lot of a Super Fresh supermarket. Dr. Osterman of the Hospital of the University of Pennsylvania performed surgery on the patient's right long, and ring fingers.

On May 12, 1987, Ms. ▮▮▮▮▮▮▮▮▮ was examined by Dr. ▮▮▮▮▮▮. She stated that she continued to have weakness of the right hand and numbness during work. She stated that she woke up several times each night with numbness in her right hand. She also reported color changes in the right hand. An EMG was performed on 8/18/87 at the Hand Rehabilitation Center and revealed a right brachial plexus neuropathy and boarder line right carpal tunnel neuropathy.

The patient participated in therapy at the Hand Rehabilitation Center for treatment of the brachial plexus neuropathy and carpal tunnel neuropathy. She had also received therapy for her initial injury at a physical therapy facility in King of Prussia. At the present time, she is discharged from therapy.

Ms. ▮▮▮▮▮▮▮▮ indicates that she has limitations in use of the right hand which includes performing activities that aggravate the right hand such as opening containers, reaching into cabinets, using a blow dryer for styling her hair, shampooing her hair, sweeping, mopping, vacuuming, writing, performing work activities as an assistant manager in a restaurant, and bowling. Ms. Harkinson indicates her major difficulties with her right upper extremity include coldness of the right long and ring fingers both indoors and outdoors, numbness in the whole right hand occurs occasionally, muscle spasms in the right arm, and pins/needles sensations in the right arm. There is no additional medical history and the patient is not taking any medications at this time.

JOB HISTORY:

Ms. ▮▮▮▮▮▮▮▮ is a student at this time. She plans to work as a lawyer when she graduates. Since she was 14, she has worked in a family owned restaurant. She describes her job requirements of restaurant work as: Lifting baskets of fried food, preparation work including cutting up vegetables for salads, dipping seafood in batter, lifting cases of canned food, and other duties include cleaning, scrubbing, hostess work, waiting on tables, cashier, and answering the phones. She stated she has difficulty at this time lifting baskets of fried food, performing preparation work, lifting cases of food (which may weight up to 60 lbs.), and lifting food trays. She states she uses her left hand for holding the phone and lifting food trays.

The Physical Capacity Evaluation consists of three components: a hand function evaluation, administration of standardized tests, and observation of performance of physical demands and job simulation.

HAND FUNCTION EVALUATION:

Grip strength taken on the Jamar Dynamometer is as follows:

Jamar Dynamometer	Right Hand		Left Hand	
Level I (tight grip)	53	lbs.	45	lbs.
Level II	78	lbs.	76	lbs.
Level III	80	lbs.	75	lbs.
Level IV	65	lbs.	65	lbs.
Level V (wide grip)	62	lbs.	65	lbs.

The Valpar Whole Body Range of Motion Work Sample was utilized to assess the patient's ability to handle and manipulate objects while working in various body positions including bending, kneeling, and stooping, using both hands, with vision partially occluded. Ms. ███ scored in the 60 percentile using the Valpar San Diego Employed Worker Norms. This score is a below average score as compared to employed worker norms from 0 to 100%.

OBSERVATION OF PERFORMANCE OF PHYSICAL DEMANDS OF WORK:

Physical Task and Observation:

1. Lifting/Carrying

Ms. ███ was able to lift and carry 20 lbs. with her right arm, and 35 lbs. with her left arm over a distance of 25 ft. She was able to lift and carry 40 lbs. with both arms.

2. Reaching

Ms. ███ was able to reach forward, overhead, and to floor level with her left arm without difficulty. When she used her right arm for reaching overhead, she reported numbness in the IV and V fingers, and in her right forearm. Endurance was poor in the right arm for reaching overhead.

3. Grasping/Handling

Ms. ███ can use her right hand for grasping and handling light sized objects without difficulty. She experienced difficulty grasping and handling small or heavy sized objects with her right hand. She can utilize her left hand for grasping and handling of small, light, and heavy sized objects without difficulty. It was observed and the patient also reported that she frequently now uses her left hand to perform most of the tasks that require grasping and handling rather than use her right hand.

4. Manipulation

Fine manipulation was below normal limits for the right and left hands.

5. Standing, Sitting, Walking

Standing tolerance is estimated by the patient to be 14 hours. Walking tolerance is estimated to be 5 miles. Sitting tolerance is estimated to be 4 hours. There was normal gait and body posture observed.

Pinch measurements were recorded with the Pinch Gauge as follows:

Pinch	Right Hand	Left Hand
Lateral Pinch:	21 lbs.	18 lbs.
3-Point Pinch:	17 lbs.	18 lbs.
Tip Pinch:		
Thumb/Index	14 lbs.	14 lbs.
Thumb/Long	9 lbs.	13 lbs.
Thumb/Ring	8 lbs.	6 lbs.
Thumb/Little	9 lbs.	8 lbs.

Active range of motion measurements were recorded with a Goniometer. The patient demonstrated full active range of motion of all joints of both her right and left upper extremities.

Volumetric measurements taken before and after the Physical Capacity Evaluation demonstrated that there was not a significant increase in hand volume in either the right and left hand after 3 hours of manual work. This indicates that this patient tolerated 3 hours of manual work without swelling occurring in either hand. Right hand volume was slightly elevated as compared to the left hand. Right hand volume measured 440 ml. as compared to 425 ml. in the left hand initially. After 3 hours of manual work, the right hand demonstrated 440 ml. and the left hand demonstrated 430 ml.

Sensibility evaluation was performed to assess Ms. ███'s light touch deep pressure and discrimanative sensation. She demonstrated diminished light touch sensation on the volar surface (palmar surface) of the right long fingertip. All other areas of both hands demonstrated normal light touch, deep pressure, and 2-point discrimination.

ADMINISTRATION OF STANDARDIZED TEST:

The Valpar Upper Extremity Range of Motion Work Sample was utilized to assess the reaching, handling, and manipulating ability of each hand. This test was performed in a confined space and with vision occluded. Ms. ███ scored in the 55 percentile using the Valpar San Diego Employed Worker Norms for the dominant right hand. She scored in the 50 percentile using the Valpar San Diego Employed Worker Norms for the non dominant left hand. These scores are both below average as employed worker norms range from 0 to 100%. The Valpar Corporation recommends that a person must score above 70% in order to performs these physical demands competitively in a work situation.

128

6. **Climbing Stairs**

Ms. ▬ was able to climb stairs without difficulty.

7. **Kneeling, Crouching, Stooping**

Ms. ▬ was able to kneel, crouch, and stoop without difficulty.

8. **Endurance**

Endurance was tested using the Work Simulator. It is a computerized evaluation instrument that can measure the amount of power emitted by the hands and arms with a variety of tools. The test compares tool use between hands for 3 minutes. On the tool simulating pushing/pulling objects, the patient's left hand demonstrated 19% more endurance than her right hand. On the tool simulating repetitive turning of a screwdriver, the patient's left hand demonstrated 29% more endurance than her right hand. On the tool simulating reaching, grasping, and pulling such as ladder climbing, the patient's left hand demonstrated 7% more endurance than her right hand. On the tool simulating repetitive gripping of pliers, the patient's right hand demonstrated 27% more endurance than her left hand.

9. **Evaluation of Consistent Effort**

Sequential testing was performed on the Work Simulator. According to the research by Vermette and Berlin (1985), on sequential tests, the coefficient of variance should be less than 15% for adult females. Ms. ▬ scored a 3.5% coefficient of variance with her right hand and a 9.0% coefficient of variance with her left hand. This indicates that the patient demonstrated consistent performance on sequential testing with both her injured and non-injured hands.

Grip strength was also measured sequentially on the Jamar Dynamometer on three occasions during the Physical Capacity Evaluation. According to the research of Bechtol (1954), the coefficient of variance on sequential grip tests should be less than 10%. Ms. ▬ scored 3.9% with her right hand and 5.9% with her left hand. This indicates consistent performance on sequential testing with both the injured and non-injured hands.

SUMMARY AND RECOMMENDATIONS:

This 21 year old, right hand dominant student has participated in treatment for a crush injury to her right long and ring fingers. She has also been treated for brachial plexus neuropathy and right carpal tunnel neuropathy. She is discharged from therapy at this time. However, the patient continues to perform a home program of exercises to control the brachial plexus neuropathy symptoms in her right upper extremity. She reported that she continues to experience numbness, tingling, and cold intolerance which are related to the brachial plexus neuropathy. The patient also reports some decreased sensation in the right long finger which was verified on the sensibility evaluation during the examination.

The patient complained of weakness and fatigue of the right upper extremity. On standardized coordination tests which required 20 to 30 minutes to complete, the patient demonstrated slow speed of coordination compared to the uninjured population. She also demonstrated decreased endurance of the right hand compared to the left hand on 3 out of the 4 tests utilized on the Work Simulator. The patient's maximum grip strength was 80 lbs. in the right hand compared to 76 lbs. in the left hand. However, this does not translate into functional capacity as the patient was not able to lift more weight with her right hand than her left hand. Her maximum lifting ability was restricted to 20 lbs. with the right hand as compared to 35 lbs. with the left hand. She demonstrated difficulty reaching overhead with her right arm as well as grasping, handling, and manipulating objects.

Based on the patient's tests response which were found to be consistent on sequential testing, it is recommended that this patient avoid job tasks that require repetitive use of the right arm for reaching, handling, manipulating, lifting, carrying, pushing, or pulling. She did demonstrate poor endurance in the right upper extremity. In the future, Ms. ▬ may have difficulty as a lawyer due to the prolonged writing requirements. She may require assistance by a dictating machine or a secretary in order to complete her reports. It is also recommended that she avoid working in the family owned restaurant performing job tasks such as preparing and cooking food, scrubbing, cleaning, or lifting food trays. She may cashier or work as a hostess. It is recommended that this patient continue to perform her home program of exercises to control symptoms of the brachial plexus neuropathy.

Patricia Baxter, MS, OTR/L

PATRICIA BAXTER, MS, OTR/L

OCCUPATIONAL THERAPY
INDIVIDUAL EVALUATION

NAME: ********************

HOME: ****** *********
     ****** *********

DOB: 04/14/59   AGE: 29

SSN: 438-19-4716

HEIGHT: 5'6"   WEIGHT: 124 lbs.

DIAGNOSIS:
1. Moderate Mental Retardation
2. Dysarthric Speech
3. Myopia
4. Hypothyrodism (mild)

DURABLE MEDICAL EQUIPMENT:
1. None
2.
3.

APPLIANCES:
1. None
2.
3.

ORTHOTICS:
1. Prescribed Glasses
2.

PROSTHETICS:
1. None
2.

ORO-MOTOR FUNCTION:

	ABSENT	IMPAIRED	PRESENT
GAG			X
SUCK			X
CHEW			X
SWALLOW			X
LIP CLOSURE			X
TONGUE			
LATERALLY			X
DEPRESS			X
ELEVATE			X
THRUST	X		

SELF-CARE:

	IND.	MIN.	MOD.	MAX.	UNABLE
HYGIENE	X				
DRESSING	X				
GROOMING	X				
FEEDING	X				
TOILETING	X				

AMOUNT OF ASSIST NEEDED

DOMESTIC SKILLS: AMOUNT OF ASSIST NEEDED

	IND.	MIN.	MOD.	MAX.	UNABLE
LAUNDRY	X				
MEAL PREP	X				
CLEANING					
ANS. PHONE	X				
ANS. DOOR	X				
SHOP		X			

COMMUNICATION
COMMUNICATION BOARD N/A
WRITE Simple
SPEAK Able
READ Simple

PERCEPTUAL
VISUAL, Within Normal Limits
MOTOR Within Normal Limits

POSTURE Within Normal Limits

HAND FUNCTION
DOMINANCE Right
GRASP PATTERN Normal
STRENGTH
NORM RT 120.8 pf   LT 110.5 pf
ACTUAL 29 pf   30 pf
VAR. S.D. 23.0 pf   16.2 pf

AMBULATION
DME REQUIRED None

TRANSFER ABILITY
TO/FROM BED Within Normal Limits
CHAIR Within Normal Limits
CAR Within Normal Limits
TOILET Within Normal Limits

JOINT RANGE OF MOTION:

TRUNK Fair to Good

LOWER EXTREMITY
HIP Fair to Good
KNEES Within Normal Limits
ANKLES Within Normal Limits

UPPER EXTREMITY
SHOULDERS Within Normal Limits
ELBOW Within Normal Limits
WRIST Within Normal Limits
FINGERS Within Normal Limits

BALANCE:
SITTING Within Normal Limits
STANDING Within Normal Limits

SENSORY Within Normal Limits

MUSCLE TONE

HYPERTONIC Minimal in Left Hamstrings and Adductors

HYPOTONIC Absent

NORMAL, Present (to low)

MOTOR PLANNING Within Normal Range

PATHOLOGICAL REFLEX None

DEFORMITIES: None

OCCUPATIONAL THERAPY

ASSESSMENT

1. Short but adequate attention span.
2. Adequate hand strength for ADL.
3. Independent in self-care.
4. Nees only further training in domestic skills.
5.
6.

RECOMMENDATIONS

1. None.
2.
3.
4.
5.
6.

PLAN

1. Hand strengthening exercises at reinforcement level.
2. Annual Occupational Therapy Evaluation.
3.
4.
5.
6.

SUSAN L. SMITH, LOTR   M.D.
10 / 17 / 88   / /

129

OCCUPATIONAL THERAPY
INDIVIDUAL EVALUATION

NAME: _____   DOB: 04/14/59   AGE: 32

HOME: _____   SSN: 438-19-4716

HEIGHT: 5'6 3/4"   WEIGHT: 116

DIAGNOSIS: 1.Mental Retardation: Moderate
2.Dysarthric Speech
3. Hypothyrodism (mild)
4. Myopia

DURABLE MEDICAL EQUIPMENT:
1. None
2.
3.

APPLIANCES:
1. Prescribed Glasses
2.
3.

ORTHOTICS:
1. None
2.

PROSTHETICS:
1. None
2.

ORO-MOTOR FUNCTION:

	ABSENT	IMPAIRED	PRESENT
GAG			X
SUCK			X
CHEW			X
SWALLOW			X
LIP CLOSURE			X
TONGUE			
LATERALLY			X
DEPRESS			X
ELEVATE			X
THRUST	X		

SELF-CARE: AMOUNT OF ASSIST NEEDED

	IND.	MIN.	MOD.	MAX.	UNABLE
HYGIENE	X				
DRESSING	X				
GROOMING	X				
FEEDING	X				
TOILETING	X				

DOMESTIC SKILLS: AMOUNT OF ASSIST NEEDED

	IND.	MIN.	MOD.	MAX.	UNABLE
LAUNDRY	X				
MEAL PREP			X		
CLEANING		X			
ANS. PHONE	X				
ANS. DOOR	X				
SHOP		X			

COMMUNICATION
COMMUNICATION BOARD N/A
WRITE Prints:Name,Address:Able to Copy
SPEAK Understandable-Fair Articulation
READ Unable

PERCEPTUAL
VISUAL Within Functional Limits
MOTOR Within Functional Limits

POSTURE Within Normal Limits

HAND FUNCTION
DOMINANCE Right
GRASP PATTERN Normal
STRENGTH
NORM Rt 121.8 pf   LT 110.4 pf
ACTUAL 40 pf   40 pf
VAR. S.D. 22.4 pf   21.7 pf

AMBULATION
DME REQUIRED None

TRANSFER ABILITY
TO/FROM BED Independent
CHAIR Independent
CAR Independent
TOILET Independent

RESIDENT: *************   IDT DATE _____   RECORD

OCCUPATIONAL THERAPY EVALUATION:

***** has a short attention span but this has been seen to improve in this past year. He is friendly and conversant. **** has worked on improving his hand grasp strength this past year and has had about a 10 psi gain in both hands. Although this is not a normal hand strength it is now adequate for light daily life tasks. *** has some limitations in daily life tasks but only needs supervision and further training.

SERVICE PLAN
1. Hand strengthening exercises at reinforcement level.
2. Annual Occupational Therapy Evaluation.

STRENGTHS
1. Pleasant personality.
2. No physical deformities or gross limitations.
3. Moderately good level of independence.

NEEDS
1. Hand strengthening exercises at a reinforcement level only.
2. Annual Occupational Therapy Evaluation.

RECOMMENDATIONS
1. None.

130